YOUR THYROID: A HOME REFERENCE

YOUR QUESTIONS. YOUR CONCERNS. YOUR RIGHT TO GOOD HEALTH.

We have written this book to help our readers identify previously unrecognized thyroid problems in themselves or among their relatives and friends. For some, it may serve as a guide to proper medical attention and treatment. We hope other readers will simply enjoy it as an introduction to a fascinating part of the remarkable body in which we live.

We have also written this book in the hope that it will reflect a new and refreshing attitude toward medical care in general. You as a patient have the *right* as well as the responsibility to know what is going on when you get sick—to know the cause of your illness, what tests or treatments you should have, why they are necessary, and what the course of your illness is likely to be. Health education of this type is important because it enables you to play a more helpful part in the care of your own body, and that in itself should help you to be a healthier person.

Your Thyroid

A Home Reference

Lawrence C. Wood, M.D., F.A.C.P.
David S. Cooper, M.D., F.A.C.P.
E. Chester Ridgway, M.D., F.A.C.P.

BALLANTINE BOOKS • NEW YORK

Library of Congress Catalog Card Number: 82-6494

ISBN 0-345-33447-7

Manufactured in the United States of America

First Ballantine Books Edition: December 1986

We dedicate this second edition of Your Thyroid *to thyroid patients and those who care for them.*

Contents

We Wrote This Book for You—

—if you are struggling with an over- or underactive thyroid and don't know it. There are two million such people in the United States alone and there are good treatments for both conditions when they are recognized.

—if any of your close relatives have a goiter or have been treated for thyroid disorders, because *many* thyroid problems run in families, and maybe you should be checked too.

—if you have an overactive thyroid, because you may have older relatives who have a failing thyroid. Some of them, as well as certain of the younger members of your family, should have their thyroids tested.

—you had neck irradiation in childhood during x-ray treatment for a condition such as acne, tonsillitis, or an enlarged thymus gland. Your risk for benign and cancerous thyroid tumors is increased (most thyroid cancers can be cured).

—if you were treated for a thyroid problem in the past and thought it was over and done with. We now know that many thyroid problems need lifelong attention.

—if you are taking thyroid pills for overweight, infertility, sluggishness, or depression, because your treatment probably needs to be reviewed and updated.

—if you are facing a test, a medical treatment, or an operation for your thyroid and want to know what it means or what it will be like.

—if you are taking or thinking of taking kelp. The iodine in kelp could make a lumpy thyroid dangerously overactive. If you are pregnant, it could make your unborn baby's thyroid enlarge or fail.

—if you are concerned about the possibility of a nuclear accident occurring near your home. There is radioactive iodine in fallout that could have harmful effects on your thyroid unless you take a small amount of nonradioactive iodine to protect your thyroid.

—if you take insulin for diabetes, need Vitamin B_{12} for anemia, have prematurely gray hair, or have white skin patches known as vitiligo. Your risk for an over- or underactive thyroid may be increased and perhaps your thyroid should be checked.

Most physicians witness the value of good patient education long before they have completed their formal medical training. It might be said that a girl named Barbara had a lot to do with the beginnings of this book. She arrived one night on the medical service at the Hospital of the University of Pennsylvania when L. C. W. was a young intern. She was seriously ill with uncontrolled diabetes—a condition known as *ketoacidosis*. During that first night of treatment, Barbara's understanding of her medical condition was impressive, and the benefits of that understanding were obvious. Her knowledge about diabetes had helped her to *do the right things at home* to control her blood sugar as she began to get sick.

It also made her aware of her limitations and told her *when to come to the hospital* as the condition worsened. In the hospital, *she was not anxious about her illness* because she knew what to expect as her treatment continued. Instead, *she was prepared to participate in her treatment*. She related a clear history of the events leading to her present problem, knew the names and dosages of her medications and the details of her diet, and was familiar with the diabetic complications that she had experienced. Finally, her understanding of her condition *prepared her to learn more about diabetes* while she was in the hospital, knowledge that would help her manage her health better in the future. Barbara had learned about her condition, in part, from talking with her physicians. But some of Barbara's understanding of her disease had come from reading *How to Live with Diabetes*, a book written for diabetic patients by Henry Dolger, M.D., and Bernard Seeman.

Recently, we three, practicing together in the Thyroid Unit of the Massachusetts General Hospital, discovered a mutual interest in patient education and a desire to write a similar book for thyroid patients. As such, it is intended for people who know they have a thyroid problem and who can use it to review and expand upon information given to them by their physicians about their condition. However, we hope this book will reach a wider audience, for many people have thyroid conditions that have not yet been recognized. Unlike diabetes, which usually makes a patient noticeably sick from the start of the illness, thyroid conditions usually begin gradually and may remain unnoticed for months or years. We hope this book will help some of our readers to identify previously unrecognized thyroid problems in themselves or among their relatives and friends and will serve as their guide toward proper medical attention and treatment. We hope other readers will simply enjoy it as an introduction to a fascinating part of the remarkable body in which we live.

We greatly appreciate the help of a large number of patients and friends who have made this book possible by their financial support through the Thyroid Clinical Research Fund at the Massachusetts General Hospital. Patients, too, have contributed meaningfully in other ways, for they teach us much about thyroid and related problems by observing their own conditions and relating these observations to us. We especially appreciate those patients who have permitted us to include their pictures to illustrate particular aspects of thyroid disease, as well as those who have written accounts of their personal experiences with thyroid problems. We feel that such accounts, which communicate a sense of the way people *feel* during thyroid illnesses, may have special meaning for others with similar problems.

We are particularly grateful to our colleagues in the thyroid field who have reviewed portions of this book and given us helpful advice pertaining to their areas of expertise. They include Doctors Gerard Burrow, David Becker, Earle Chapman, John Crawford, Delbert Fisher, William Green, Alvin Hayles, Sidney Ingbar, Farahe Maloof, Edward Rose, Paul Walfish, and Robert Volpé. In a similar way we appreciate the help and comments of family members as well as close personal friends, many of whom have thyroid problems or related conditions. They have given us valuable criticism periodically during numerous manuscript revisions.

We would also like to acknowledge the artistic contributions of Linda Hoffman-Kimball and Alex Gray. Linda's creative drawings highlight the text in many special ways, while Alex's medical illustrations clarify many aspects of thyroid anatomy and function.

We appreciate the friendship and good working relationships that we have enjoyed with our publishing staff at Houghton Mifflin and especially with our capable editors, Ruth Hapgood and Lois Randall. We also are indebted to Ruth DiBlasi, Kelly Gritz, Dianna Lynch, and Sharon Melanson for skilled clerical assistance.

Preface to the Second Edition of *Your Thyroid: A Home Reference*

We are pleased that the success of the first edition of *Your Thyroid* has led to publication of a revised edition in this new form, and hope that it will continue to be meaningful and helpful to patients, to those who care for them, and to the general public.

We are thankful to Marilyn Abraham and Sheila Curry at Ballantine Books for their expert editorial advice, and to Connie Clausen for her direction and encouragement and for facilitating our association with Ballantine. We welcome the new artwork by Karen Dardinski and Anita Karl. We also are grateful to Ruth Hapgood, our former editor and now a close friend, for help with this revision of the text.

Most of all we thank the patients, physicians, and other interested readers who took the time to write us about the first edition. We have heeded their comments and suggestions and hope that they will be pleased with this new volume.

CHAPTER ONE

Why We Wrote This Book

Thyroid troubles are common, affecting human beings everywhere. The World Health Organization estimates that 200 million people have enlarged thyroids known as *goiters*. Autopsy studies in the United States reveal that about half of the population have lumps or nodules in their thyroid glands, and random surveys suggest that sometime in our lives, between 5 and 10 percent of us will develop a thyroid nodule big enough to be found by a physician during a routine medical checkup.

Even more surprising, and probably of greater importance, are recent findings regarding the prevalence of disorders of thyroid function: overactive thyroids (hyperthyroidism) and underactive thyroids (hypothyroidism). In the United States, reports have appeared since 1978 from Connecticut, Massachusetts, and California suggesting that there may be nearly ten million Americans whose thyroid glands are now either overactive or underactive. More important, nearly two million of them do not even know they are sick.[1] Even among those who know they have a thyroid condition, many are taking too much or too little medication and need an examination and readjustment of their treatment.

Just like anyone else, you could have a thyroid problem. And yet, you may know so little about the thryoid that you don't even suspect it as the culprit when you feel sick. But if you go to your doctor feeling sluggish, cold, and tired, one of the things that he or she will consider is whether your thyroid gland is underactive. On the other hand, if you feel that your "engine is racing," your pulse rate is rapid, and you can't seem to slow down, your thyroid may be overstimulating your system. If the lower part of your neck is swollen, you may have a *goiter*, often the first sign that your thyroid is beginning to malfunction. If you have a sore throat and ache all over so that you're sure you have "flu," it is possible that you have an inflammation of your thyroid known as *subacute thyroiditis*. If you are washing or shaving one morning and happen to feel a lump in the front of your neck, it may be a *cyst* or *tumor* in your thyroid.

You don't have to live with these conditions; they can be helped, and often very easily. For example, changes in the level of thyroid function can be treated with medication, and the inflammation of thyroiditis is often controlled by aspirin alone. Simple tests on a thyroid nodule can tell not only what kind of lump it is, but also whether it should be operated upon, treated with medication, or perhaps just left alone.

On the other hand, perhaps you had a thyroid problem in the past. If so, it is important to realize a fact that we did not know thirty years ago: Often thyroid troubles are not permanently cured. For example, there seems to be a natural tendency for most patients with hyperthyroidism to progress toward hypothyroidism in later years. Thus, if you had an overactive thyroid in 1950, even though you were "cured" then and have had many healthy years since that time, you may now have a failing thyroid gland. In 1950 we did not know that late thyroid failure was common among patients who had an overactive gland earlier in life, so you and others like you not told to have periodic thyroid checkups for the rest of your lives. In addition, you may have changed physicians since then and your new doctor may not even be aware of your earlier thyroid problems. If this is your situation, you can help yourself by learning about the symptoms of a failing thyroid gland and by telling your physician about your past thyroid disorder. If your thyroid level proves to be low, it can be corrected simply by taking a thyroid hormone tablet once a day.

Another consideration in the detection of thyroid trouble is that certain problems tend to happen to more than one member of a family because the conditions are inherited. Thus, a young woman of twenty-three who is now ill with hyperthyroidism may have a parent or grandparent whose thyroid gland has been overactive and is now underactive. Possibly, he or she never was obviously hyperthyroid, but still may be hypothyroid now. That older relative may think that his or her sluggishness, constipation, lack of pep, and dislike for cold weather are simply signs of old age. Instead, they could well be *treatable* symptoms of hypothyroidism.

There are several medical conditions that are common in patients who have certain thyroid diseases. Some, like early graying of the hair, are familiar and do not need treatment. Others, like the white spots or white skin patches of *vitiligo* and the blood condition known as *pernicious anemia*, may be unfamiliar to you or other members of your family. This book will help you to recognize such associated conditions and will also describe how many of them can be treated.

For example, if someone in your family has had an overactive or underactive thyroid, you and some of your relatives may develop pernicious anemia as well. This blood disorder appears if you become unable to absorb Vitamin B_{12} from food. Unfortunately, it can begin so gradually that the problem may not be recognized for years, during which you may feel sick with fatigue, have numb hands and feet, and perhaps even have mental changes that are mistaken for "old age." Yet these symptoms can be relieved and even prevented from occurring by the timely administration of Vitamin B_{12}.

We have written this book to explain these common problems to you if you have one of these conditions. We have also written it in the hope that it will reflect a new and refreshing attitude toward medical care in general. You as a patient have the *right* as well as the *responsibility* to know what is going on when you get sick—to know the cause of your illness, what tests and treatments you should have, why those tests and treatments are necessary, and what the course of your illness is likely to be. Health education of this type is important because it enables you to play a more helpful part in the care of your own body, and that in itself should help you to be a healthier person.

CHAPTER TWO

General Information

Normal and Abnormal Thyroid Function, Thyroid Diseases, Thyroid Tests, and Thyroid Treatments

Your Thyroid is one of the many glands in your body that make special chemicals known as *hormones*. Hormones travel in your blood stream throughout your body to affect many different parts of your system, including your brain, heart, liver, kidneys, and skin. Therefore, it is not surprising that a change in any hormone level can produce abnormalities all over your body. The particular hormone made by your thyroid gland acts on these receptors somehow to affect the *rate* at which many bodily processes happen.

Normally, your blood level of thyroid hormone is constant, with little day-to-day variation. However, if the gland becomes diseased, it may produce *high* thyroid hormone levels that may speed up body processes, causing symptoms like rapid heartbeat (palpitations), nervousness, frequent bowel movements, and weight loss as you burn up calories more rapidly. In contrast, a poorly functioning gland may produce *less* than a normal amount of thyroid hormone, which may slow your heartbeat and make you tired and constipated. A low thyroid hormone level also may cause your skin, hair, and fingernails to grow more slowly, so they become rough, dry, and brittle. You may gain a little weight, though you are unlikely to become really fat. In short, if your thyroid is underactive, you will probably feel generally "rundown."

Your thyroid is normally found in the front of your neck (Figure 1). Its two halves or *lobes* normally weigh about one ounce. They lie on either side of your windpipe, just below your "Adam's apple," and are joined together by a narrow band of thyroid tissue known as the *isthmus*. Occasionally, a small amount of thyroid tissue will project upward from the isthmus along your windpipe. This tissue, called the *pyramidal lobe*, is a reminder that, before you were born, your thyroid migrated from its place of origin at the back of your tongue down to the front of your neck.

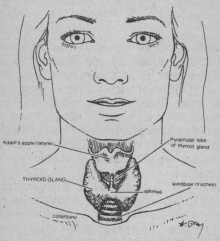

Figure 1 Your thyroid gland is normally located in the front of your neck below your Adam's apple.

HOW THE THYROID WORKS

Iodine is found in many foods, especially seafood, salt, bread, and milk. The thyroid takes this dietary iodine from your blood stream and uses it to make thyroid hormones (Figure 2). The two most important of these hormones are triiodothyronine (T_3) and thryoxine (T_4). (The nicknames "T_3" and "T_4" refer to the number of iodine atoms contained in each hormone molecule: There are three iodine atoms in T_3 and four in T_4.) These hormones are stored within your thyroid until they are needed, when they are released into your blood stream and transported throughout your body attached to special *carrier proteins*. After entering the cells of your body tissues, they go into *nuclei* at the center of each cell, where they attach to specific *receptors* (Figure 3). Despite our knowledge of how thyroid hormones look and where they work in your body, we still have very little understanding of how they *act* on these receptors to regulate the various activities of your body tissues.

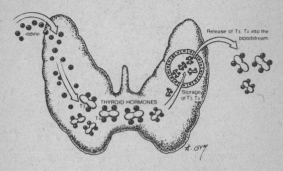

Figure 2 Manufacture, storage, and release of thyroid hormones.

Although your thyroid has some inherent ability to produce thyroid hormone by itself, its function is governed largely by the pituitary gland, located at the base of your brain. When your level of thyroid hormone falls too low, the pituitary responds by producing *thyroid stimulating hormone* (TSH). If your thyroid is healthy, it responds to TSH by working harder, thereby raising the blood level of thyroid hormone back to normal.

Several factors seem to influence the way the pituitary gland controls thyroid function. A low blood level of thyroid hormone, for example, appears to influence the pituitary gland directly, provoking an increase in TSH release. On the other hand, the pituitary is itself under the control of still higher centers in the brain, including the *hypothalamus* and the *cerebral cortex* (Figure 3). The interactions between these higher centers of the brain and the thyroid are currently under careful study by research workers.

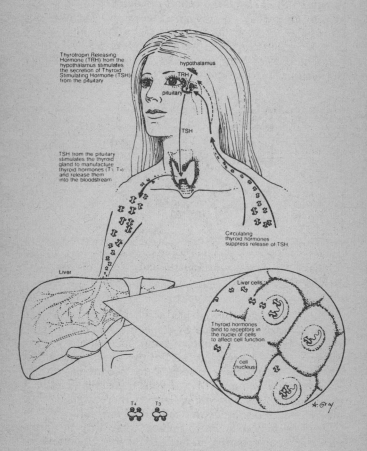

Figure 3   The Hypothalamic-Pituitary-Thyroid Axis.

FACTORS INVOLVED IN THYROID DISEASES

Various things can go wrong with your thyroid gland: It can produce too much hormone (*hyper*thyroidism) or too little (*hypo*thyroidism); it can become infected or inflamed (*thyroiditis*), or it can develop a cyst or a tumor. Perhaps the most common thyroid abnormality is a *goiter*, a simple enlargement of the thyroid gland itself. More than one of these conditions may exist or develop with time in a single patient, and different but related thyroid abnormalities may occur in several members of the same family. Although research workers still do not understand all of the mechanisms that produce thyroid disease, we do know a lot about some of the factors involved.

Genetics

The tendency to develop some thyroid problems appears to be inherited. The best studied of these conditions are some rare disorders that result from a failure in the production of thyroid hormone. In some of these disorders, the thyroid has difficulty getting enough iodine from the blood stream. In others, there is a problem with the use of the iodine to make the more complex thyroid hormone molecules.

Heredity also appears to have a role in most instances in which the thyroid changes its level of function and become either overactive or underactive. Yet, even those who have inherited the *tendency* to develop one of these thyroid conditions may never become ill. Therefore, thyroid disease within a family may seem to "skip" generations: You may have a thyroid problem, and, though your parents seem healthy, you may learn of a grandparent who had thyroid trouble, too. In other instances, several different thyroid problems will show up in one family: Some relatives may develop overactive thyroids and others may develop underactive thyroids; some may become very sick, while others may be only mildly affected.

Sex

Virtually all thyroid disorders appear to be more common in women than in men. Hyperthyroidism, for example, occurs seven to nine times more commonly in women than in men. As of now, we don't know why women have this unusual tendency.

Age

If your thyroid is going to become overactive, you are most likely to be somewhere between the ages of twenty and forty when it happens. On the other hand, if your thyroid fails, it will be more likely to do so at a much later age—probably after you reach fifty years of age. Similarly, certain types of thyroid tumors tend to occur in young people while others are more common in older individuals.

Diet

Despite the efforts of many health organizations, there are still many people in the world (especially in remote mountainous areas) who do not get enough iodine in their diets. As a result, they have an increased tendency to develop goiters and serious hypothyroidism. In America, on the other hand, iodine deficiency does not exist. Our problem is the opposite: Our diets contain a more than adequate supply of iodine, and we may get even more in medicines, health foods, or dyes that are used to x-ray our kidneys, gall bladder, or spinal canal. Too much iodine can abruptly raise or lower thyroid activity in some people with underlying thyroid disease, but fortunately, most of us are unaffected when we are exposed to excessive amounts of iodine. (See Chapter 14 for further information about this public health problem.)

Some foods contain *goitrogens*, chemicals that can cause goiter by interfering with thyroid hormone production. Such foods include cabbage, kale, rutabaga, and turnips. Fortunately, the amount of goitrogen in these foods is so low that it would take vast quantities of one or more of them to cause a significant change in thyroid function. Soybean extracts are also capable of producing thyroid enlargement by decreasing the amount of iodine that is absorbed from the intestine. In the 1950s, for example, soy protein was found to be the cause of goiter and iodine deficiency in infants who were fed soy formula instead of milk because of milk allergy. This problem was corrected simply by adding some iodine to the soy formula. Soy protein is now being used in increasing quantities in adult foods as an inexpensive source of protein. At present there is no evidence that it is doing us any harm, probably because of the abundance of iodine in our diets.

Medication

Sometimes a medication will change thyroid function. For example, lithium, a drug used to treat certain psychiatric disorders, can cause both goiter and hypothyroidism in some people. Governmental agencies carefully test new drugs for side effects, and if you are given a drug that can harm your thyroid, you will probably be warned about it by your physician or your pharmacist, or by reading the label on the medicine bottle.

Radiation

You are being exposed continuously to small amounts of environmental radiation. There is no evidence that the amount of radiation that your thyroid receives in this manner is harmful. On the other hand, if you have a tumor or other medical condition near your thyroid gland that must be treated with a larger dose of x-rays, or if your thyroid is exposed to a relatively large amount of environmental radiation (as it might be in a nuclear accident or explosion), it may be seriously affected. Your thyroid may become underactive, but this problem can be corrected if you take thyroid hormone tablets. The greater concern about radiation exposure is that thyroid cancer could develop. We now know that people who are given radiation treatments to the thyroid area have an increased risk for developing thyroid nodules in the years that follow. Some of these nodules may contain thyroid cancer (see Chapter 12).

Stress

Stress represents an additional environmental problem, but one that is hard to evaluate. Most physicians who see a lot of patients with thyroid dysfunction are impressed by the fact that the commonest form of hyperthyroidism often follows a period of life stress, particularly a loss such as a death in the family or the loss of a job. Some recent studies suggest that stress can alter the immune system which in turn may cause changes in thyroid function. In spite of these apparent associations, we still do not know exactly *how* stress influences your thyroid, or why such stressful situations appear to affect the thyroids of some people more than others.

Infections

Bacterial infections of the thyroid are very rare. Infections due to viruses (such as those that produce the common cold) are more likely to cause thyroid disease, and are thought to do so in a disorder called subacute thyroiditis.

THYROID TESTS

Highly sensitive and specific methods are now available to measure the blood levels of the thyroid hormones, *thyroxine* (T_4) and *triiodothyroxine* (T_3), as well as the concentration of the pituitary hormone, *thyroid stimulating hormone* (TSH). These tests have almost entirely supplanted the previously used but less precise tests of *basal metabolic rate* and *protein-bound iodine*. Measurements of T_4 and TSH are the most important tests that physicians perform today to determine the *function* of the thyroid gland.

Other thyroid blood tests are used to evaluate a phenomenon known as *protein binding of thyroid hormone*. Some thyroid hormone travels in your blood stream in a "free" or active form, but most (greater that 99 percent) is in a "bound" or inactive form that is held by a chemical attraction to certain proteins in your blood. Only the free form of the hormone can act within your body cells. Factors like pregnancy or medications may alter the amount of bound hormone, but the free level remains normal so you feel well. In order to estimate the amount of free active hormone, a blood test called the *T_3 resin uptake* is used. This is an inexpensive, indirect method of estimating the proportions of active and inactive hormone. When more precise information is required, it is also possible to measure your blood level of free thyroid hormone directly, as well as the concentrations of the thyroid binding proteins themselves.

One of the most important advances in thyroid research came in the late 1930s, when physicians learned how to use *radioactive iodine* to study thyroid function. Since the thyroid gland uses iodine to make thyroid hormone, physicians can use radioactive iodine in several ways to diagnose and treat thyroid problems. If you have a *radioactive iodine uptake test*, you will be given a tiny amount of either radioactive iodine (^{123}Iodine is the preferred isotope), usually contained in a small capsule that is easily swallowed. The radioactive iodine (or "radioiodine") goes to your thyroid gland to be used as dietary iodine in the manufacture of thyroid hormones. Twenty-four hours later a radiation detector or *counter* held in front of your thyroid gland tells your physician the exact percentage of radioiodine that has been taken up by your thyroid. If your thyroid is overactive, it may take up nearly all of the iodine you swallowed, but if it is underactive, it will usually take up very little. If your thyroid is inflamed (thyroiditis), it also may take up very little iodine.

You may be found to have low radioiodine uptake if you are taking thyroid hormone tablets or if you have ingested excessive amounts of iodine in medicine or food (such as certain cough remedies, vitamins, and kelp). Similarly, a low radioiodine uptake will occur in the weeks following the administration of iodine-containing dyes that have been used to x-ray your kidneys, gall bladder, or other organs. Under these circumstances, the test would not reflect accurately the activity of your thyroid.

At the time of the radioiodine uptake test, your doctor also may want a picture of your thyroid gland known as a *thyroid scan*.* Here, the radiation detector in front of your neck is attached to a *scanner*, which can draw pic-

---

*In some medical centers, a radioactive substance known as technetium is used instead of radioiodine for some thyroid scans.

tures showing the pattern of radioiodine within your thyroid gland. The procedure takes just a few minutes and is done while you are lying comfortably on an examining table.

A thyroid scan may provide valuable information in a variety of situations. If your thyroid gland is overactive, the scan indicates whether the entire gland is abnormal or whether just parts of it are overactive (such areas are sometimes referred to as "hot nodules" because of their excessive activity and the picture they make in a thyroid scan). Unfortunately, a thyroid scan is not very helpful in evaluating lumps within the gland that are suspected of containing cancer. Thyroid cysts, harmless tumors, and cancers all tend to concentrate radioiodine poorly. On the other hand, if a lump within the thyroid shows a normal or increased uptake of radioiodine in the thyroid scan, that is a strong indication that the lump does not contain cancer. (Figures 4–8 are an artist's rendering of several different thyroid scan patterns.)

Your physician will always be mindful of your welfare in deciding whether to expose you to even the small amounts of radioactivity given to your thyroid and (to a far lesser degree) to the rest of your body during these tests.[3]

If more information about a thyroid nodule is needed, your physician may recommend a second type of thyroid picture, one that can be made by using sound waves in a manner similar to that of radar. In this procedure, known as a *thyroid ultrasound*, you will be asked to lie quietly while a small instrument known as a *transducer* sends sound waves through your thyroid gland. The sound waves passing through the tissue echo back to the transducer and produce a picture of your thyroid gland. Dark spaces appear where cysts are found, while solid tumors show as a different pattern of light and dark markings.

There are also occasions in which your physician may want to obtain a small sample of your thyroid tissue in order to find out whether a nodule contains thyroid cancer or to understand why your gland has enlarged. In

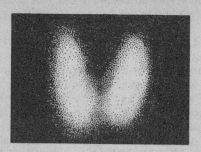

Figure 4 A normal thyroid scan.

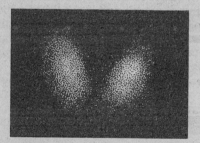

Figure 5 An underactive thyroid.

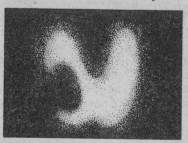

Figure 6 An inactive or "cold" nodule.

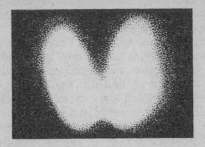

Figure 7 Overactivity of the entire thyroid.

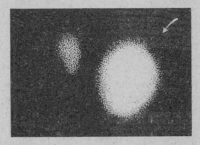

Figure 8 An overactive or "hot" nodule.

some instances, a *needle biopsy* of the thyroid can be done. In this test, after numbing the skin of your neck with a local anesthetic, the physician penetrates the thyroid with a small hollow needle through which a tiny amount of tissue can be removed for examination under a microscope. If the tissue contains cancer, removal of the nodule is necessary. Needless to say, the finding of a thyroid cyst or other harmless lump by means of a thyroid biopsy has saved many thousands of patients from unnecessary thyroid surgery. (See the discussion of a thyroid biopsy in Chapter 10.)

A variety of other tests can be used to understand specific thyroid problems. Some of these involve injections of hormones that stimulate your thyroid or pituitary gland in order to find out more about how your thyroid is working. Such tests can be particularly helpful when thyroid disease is suspected but the more conventional tests have failed to tell exactly what the problem is. These procedures will be described later in this book when we discuss their use in the evaluation of specific thyroid diseases.

THYROID TREATMENTS

If your thyroid is *overactive* and producing too much thyroid hormone, it can be controlled in three ways: medication (pills), thyroid surgery, and radioactive iodine. Some medications interrupt the manufacture of thyroid hormones, while others work by blocking the action of the hormones on body tissues. Your thyroid blood level will be reduced, of course, if a surgeon removes part of your thyroid gland, since that is where the hormone is coming from. Radioactive iodine also can be used to treat overactivity of the thyroid gland, since radiation will damage thyroid tissue and decrease hormone production.[4] The amount of radioactive iodine needed to damage thyroid tissue and thus treat hyperthyroidism is much larger than the amount used in a thyroid scan. Furthermore, we use ^{131}I, which causes more radiation effect on thyroid tissue than the less-damaging ^{123}I usually used in scans.

If your thyroid is *underactive*, thyroid hormone supplements can be given in tablet form to raise your thyroid blood level to normal. The same tablets may also be helpful in reducing the size of nodules or large goiters in some patients.

Thyroid cancers are best treated by surgery aimed at removing the entire cancer. The use of radioactive iodine can also be helpful, especially if the tumor is too widespread to be removed surgically. Finally, thyroid hormone medicine is always used to reduce the spread of a thyroid cancer that cannot be removed entirely or to prevent recurrence of a cancer that has been removed.

In summary, we understand what your thyroid gland does, we can test it very accurately and with great safety, and we can almost always tell whether you have thyroid disease and if it is mild or serious. Drugs, radioactive iodine, and surgery are available to treat thyroid disorders, and often more than one treatment can be used for the same condition. Thus, appropriate treatment can be "tailor-made" for you no matter what sort of thyroid problem you might develop.

CHAPTER THREE

Goiter

The Big Thyroid

> I've grown a goitre while living in this den, as cast from
> stagnant streams in Lombardy, or in what other land they
> hap to be.
>
> —From a sonnet written by Michelangelo while he was paint-
> ing the Sistine Chapel

The word *goiter* often frightens patients who think it
means thyroid *cancer*. Actually, the term merely means
an enlarged thyroid gland (Figure 9). There are a great
many causes of goiter, and ironically, cancer is the least
common of all.

The Chinese apparently noticed goiters around 1600
B.C., and were even aware that burned sponge and seaweed sometimes made them smaller. Although iodine
was not discovered until 1812, we now suspect that it
was iodine in the sponge and seaweed that made the Chinese goiters smaller, and that the thyroid glands had enlarged in the first place due to an insufficiency of iodine
in the diet. To the ancient Romans, when the neck of a
newly married girl swelled, it was taken as a sign that
she was pregnant. In some tribal cultures, pregnancy
was diagnosed when a goiter developed and broke a
thread necklace. Michelangelo, like others of his time,
thought that goiter happened when someone drank water
that contained something that made the neck swell. Instead, as in all of the other examples mentioned, his
goiter was probably due to iodine deficiency in the region in which he was living.

For centuries, physicians used the term *goiter* to describe almost any kind of throat swelling, not just enlargement of the thyroid. (Indeed, the word may have come from the Latin word *guttur*, which means throat.) This confused their efforts to find the causes and cures for goiters, since they applied the term to so many different conditions.

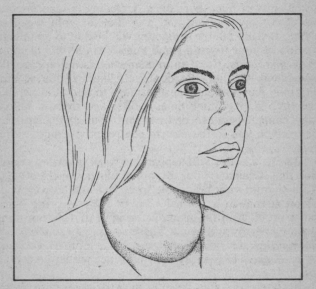

Figure 9   A patient with a goiter.

If you have a goiter and you live in the United States, the goiter is not due to iodine deficiency in your diet. This problem no longer exists in America and is rare in other developed countries. Rather, your thyroid enlargement means that something else is wrong with your thyroid gland.

The presence of a goiter may mean that your thyroid is becoming overactive. If so, you may also have other evidence of *hyper*thyroidism, such as a rapid pulse, nervousness, weight loss, diarrhea, and shaky hands. On the other hand, a goiter may be the first sign that your thyroid is failing. In that case, falling blood levels of thyroid hormone have caused your pituitary gland, located deep in your brain, to release thyroid stimulating hormone (TSH), which has caused your thyroid to grow larger. If this is your problem, you may also have other complaints of *hypo*thyroidism, including fatigue, mental dullness, constipation, and a dislike for cold weather. Often, thyroid failure and goiter will be due to an inflammation of your thyroid gland known as *chronic lymphocytic thyroiditis*. Such an inflammation is not apparently associated with an infection. Yet, like arthritis or bursitis, the reaction can cause damage to body tissues like the thyroid. At other times, goiter and thyroid failure may happen because of treatment your physician may have given you in the past to control an overactive thyroid.

Rarely, a goiter will appear due to an inherited condition that is causing your thyroid to function ineffectively. Your thyroid may be unable to collect iodine from your blood stream in a normal way, or there may be some other problem in the manufacturing of thyroid hormone within your thyroid gland. These so-called *metabolic abnormalities* are rare, but it can be helpful to you and your relatives to identify their presence within your family.

A goiter may also develop in association with an infection of your thyroid gland. If so, your thyroid will probably be very painful, and there may be other evidence of the infection, including fever, sluggishness, and aching muscles.

Sometimes what seems to be a generalized enlargement of your entire thyroid gland will prove instead to be a lump or *nodule* that has appeared within the gland. Fortunately, most of these nodules do not contain cancer but are due instead to benign (harmless) tumors, fluid-filled *cysts*, or other harmless conditions.

Finally and *most common of all*, you may develop a

goiter without any change in the activity of your thyroid, without inflammation or infection, and without evidence of a cyst or tumor. This type of thyroid enlargement has several names. Some physicians probably use the term *simple goiters* because they rarely cause complications. Others refer to them as *nontoxic goiters* because they usually don't make you sick. We prefer to call them *multinodular goiters* because they all contain many small nodules and tend to become more obviously lumpy in later years. Such goiters tend to run in families and, like most thyroid problems, are more common in women than in men. They usually function normally, but may cause hyperthyroidism, especially in elderly patients.

If you develop a goiter, you should have a thyroid evaluation, including an examination by a physician and tests of thyroid functions. This is important, because your goiter may be the first sign of a thyroid problem, and prompt evaluation and early treatment may keep you from becoming seriously sick.

During your examination, your physician will ask you about symptoms that might indicate a change in the function of your thyroid gland. He or she will also want to know whether other members of your family have had thyroid problems, for your goiter may be the first indication that you have a similar condition.

The thyroid tests that your physician chooses to help find the cause of your goiter will depend in part on what has been found during your examination. If your physician suspects an overactive or underactive thyroid, tests that measure your blood level of thyroid hormone and pituitary hormone TSH may be helpful. Blood tests may also reveal the presence of substances known as *autoantibodies* in your blood—evidence that your thyroid is affected by thyroiditis. *Radioactive scans* can help by showing the function of your entire thyroid or of nodules within your thyroid gland. An *ultrasound* thyroid picture made with sound waves can also be helpful in distinguishing between a solid thyroid nodule and a fluid-filled cyst. Finally, it is even possible that your physician will obtain a piece of your thyroid gland tissue to examine under a microscope. That procedure, known as a thyroid *biopsy*, can be especially helpful if cancer is suspected.

Since most goiters seem to work perfectly well and do not contain cancer, your physician may decide that no treatment is necessary unless your thyroid grows so big that it becomes unsightly, or causes hoarseness, difficulty in swallowing, or discomfort in your neck. In such cases you may be given thyroid hormone tablets to *suppress* the function of your pituitary gland, which normally controls your thyroid. By inhibiting the release of thyroid stimulating hormone from your pituitary gland the thyroid tablets may cause your goiter to decrease in size and thereby relieve your complaints. If the goiter does not shrink with hormone treatment it can be removed surgically, although an operation is rarely necessary. On the other hand, if tests reveal that a problem such as a medication, a change in thyroid function, or a cancer has caused your goiter, your physician will treat you for that specific problem.

In summary, if your thyroid enlarges it is probably a harmless multinodular goiter, but it may mean that something else is wrong for which you may need treatment. Therefore, you should arrange to have a medical examination and appropriate tests performed by your physician. In the following chapters we will describe in detail many of the problems that can cause goiter and abnormal thyroid function, which may be disclosed by your medical examination.

CHAPTER FOUR

The Overactive Thyroid

Hyperthyroidism Caused by Graves' Disease (Diffuse Toxic Goiter)

A lady, aged twenty, became affected with some symptoms which were supposed to be hysterical . . . After she had been in this nervous state about three months it was observed that her pulse had become singularly rapid . . . She next complained of weakness on exertion and began to look pale and thin . . . It was observed that the eyes assumed a singular appearance, for the eyeballs were apparently enlarged. In a few months . . . a tumour, of a horseshoe shape, appeared on the front of the throat and exactly in the situation of the thyroid gland.

> —From the Clinical Lectures delivered by Robert J. Graves, M.D., at the Meath Hospital in Dublin, Ireland, during the Session of 1834-5 (*London Medical and Surgical Journal* vol. 7, part 2, p. 516 [1835]).

The most common type of hyperthyroidism is produced by a generalized overactivity of the entire thyroid gland. This is called *diffuse toxic goiter*: *diffuse* because the *entire* gland is involved in the disease process, *toxic* because the patient appears hot and flushed, as if he or she were "toxic" due to an infection, and *goiter* because the overactivity enlarges the gland. Diffuse toxic goiter is also known as *Graves' disease*, in honor the Irish physician, Robert J. Graves, who was one of the first to describe this condition and who first noted the protrusion of the eyes that is sometimes associated with it.

If you develop Graves' disease, your thyroid will begin to produce more and more thyroid hormone. As it does so, the gland will usually grow larger and will, in most cases, grow big enough to protrude noticeably in the front of your neck. You may notice the enlargement in your neck yourself, or you may not notice anything until a friend or family physician points it out. If the goiter is small, you may only sense the presence of a lump while swallowing. Typically, in this form of hyperthyroidism your thyroid gland is not tender, and it is not uncomfortable when you swallow.

As you develop hyperthyroidism, you may lose weight even though you seem to eat plenty of food. You may feel nervous and jumpy and may become quite irritable and quarrelsome. You are likely to perspire more than usual and dislike hot weather. Your skin may gradually become thin and delicate, and you may notice that you are losing some of the hair on your head. As your fingernails grow more rapidly, you may notice an irregularity of the nail margin, making it difficult for you to keep your fingernails clean.

Muscle weakness, especially involving your upper arms and thighs, may make it difficult for you to carry heavy packages or to climb stairs. You may, in fact, experience such marked leg weakness that you cannot stand up from a squatting position without help. You may notice that your hands shake, and at times this tremor may become so severe that you can't even carry a cup of coffee without its rattling or spilling in its saucer. Your heartbeat may speed up from a normal rate of seventy or eighty to well over one hundred beats per minute. Occasionally, without warning, your pulse may quicken abruptly, causing very rapid palpitations that last several minutes and then end as mysteriously and abruptly as they began. You are unlikely to have real diarrhea, but your bowel movements may become loose and more frequent.

If you are a woman, your menstrual cycle may change. Your flow may become much lighter and the interval between menstrual periods may lengthen. More rarely, your periods may become irregular, or may cease entirely, making it more difficult for you to become pregnant. If pregnancy does occur, there appears to be an increased likelihood that you will have a miscarriage. Women usually notice little change in their breasts, but if you are a man, your breasts may become slightly larger and may be tender.

One of the most puzzling and least understood aspects of Graves' disease is the way it may affect your eyes. Usually the change is simply an elevation of your upper eyelids that makes your eyes appear more prominent (Figure 10). Occasionally, however, swelling of the tissue behind your eyeballs may cause actual protrusion of the eyes known as *exophthalmos*. Sometimes your eyes will feel dry or become red and irritated. A few patients have involvement of their eye muscles that may make them see double. In its most extreme (and very rare) form, the nerve to one or both of your eyes becomes inflamed and you may have trouble with your vision. This condition is known as *optic neuropathy*.

Elevation of the upper eyelids may be seen in anyone who has a high level of thyroid hormone, even someone who is taking thyroid hormone tablets in excess. The other things that can happen to your eyes in Graves' disease are unrelated to your blood level of thyroid hormone. If you are one of the people with Graves' disease who develops eye inflammation and protrusion, the eye problems probably will begin when you first become hyperthyroid. Quite often, however, eye problems and thyroid overactivity occur at different times, occasionally separated from one another by many years. Very rarely, a person may develop eye trouble as the only manifestation of Graves' disease.

Eye disease is therefore one problem that occurs only in the type of hyperthyroidism that is caused by Graves' disease. Another condition unique to Graves' disease is a skin disorder that may appear on the front of your legs and rarely on top of your feet. This is called *pretibial myxedema*,* and takes the form of a lumpy, reddish-

---

*See Chapter 9 for a more complete discussion of the eye problems and the pretibial myxedema that may occur in Graves' disease.

colored thickening of your skin. It is usually painless and not serious. As with the eye trouble in Graves' disease, pretibial myxedema may occur anytime. Its appearance does not necessarily coincide with the beginning of your thyroid problem, nor is its severity related to your blood level of thyroid hormone.

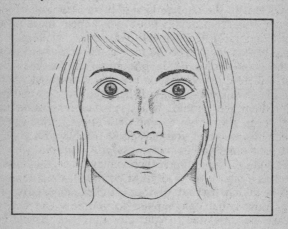

Figure 10   Eyelid elevation may be seen in any type of hyperthyroidism.

WHAT CAUSES GRAVES' DISEASE?

Graves' disease seems to be caused by the interaction of a variety of different factors, including heredity, your body's immune system, your age, sex hormones, and stress. Some sort of genetic predisposition seems to be needed first, and can be thought of as an inherited *tendency* to develop hyperthyroidism. If you have this factor, you *may* develop Graves' disease at some time during your life, or you may not, but if you lack this genetic factor, you probably cannot develop this disorder.

This type of hyperthyroidism clearly runs in families. If you have Graves' disease, and if sensitive thyroid tests could be carried out on your relatives, they might show mild thyroid abnormalities in one of your parents and one of your grandparents, as well as in some of your aunts, uncles, brothers, and sisters, and possibly in some of your children as well. Fortunately, few of these relatives will ever become sick enough from their thyroid problems to require treatment; but as we suggest in Chapter 8, some of them should be checked occasionally in this regard by their family physician.

Studies in identical twins confirm the importance of genetics in Graves' disease and also show the ability of other factors to modify the disease. Usually, identical twins either both have Graves' disease or neither develops the problem. But since other factors influence the disease process, twins rarely experience the onset of hyperthyroidism at the same time, and the *course* of the disease in the twins may be quite different.

There appear to be many different factors that can "trigger off" Graves' disease in a person who has inherited a tendency to it. Many thyroid specialists believe that *stress* can play a role in starting the hyperthyroidism, for we have all seen patients in whom a stressful situation, such as a death in the family, has preceded the onset of this condition. *Sex hormones* are also important, for the disease is seven to nine times more common in women than in men, and not infrequently begins after a hormonal change such as pregnancy. *Age* also seems to have something to do with the onset of Graves' disease, since it is most likely to appear when you are between the ages of twenty and forty. Finally, your body's *immune system* appears to play a role in the production of this disorder. By an unknown mechanism, substances called *autoantibodies* appear in your blood and stimulate the thyroid to overactivity, causing it to make more thyroid hormone. Thus, instead of being under the control of the pituitary gland, which is the normal situation, your thyroid becomes controlled by these abnormal antibodies in your blood.

In summary, a susceptible person develops Graves' disease because of one or more factors that trigger off thyroid overactivity. As thyroid function increases, more thyroid hormones are released into the blood stream, producing the symptoms of hyperthyroidism.

DIAGNOSING GRAVES' DISEASE

If you go to your doctor with symptoms that suggest an overactive thyroid, the diagnosis can usually be confirmed easily and safely. In your examination, your doctor will look for a goiter, a rapid pulse, a tremor, and other evidence of hyperthyroidism. If such evidence is found, a sample of your blood can be tested for the level of the thyroid hormone *thyroxine* (T_4). If your T_4 level is high, it confirms the presence of hyperthyroidism.*

Thyroid hormones are carried to your blood largely in an inactive form attached to certain of your blood proteins, so only a very small amount of your thyroid hormone is free and active. Pregnancy, birth control pills, and other nonthyroid factors may increase the total amount of thyroid hormone bound to protein and give a false impression of hyperthyroidism, even though your free active T_4 level remains normal. A *T_3 resin uptake* blood test is an inexpensive means of clarifying the situation by telling whether your *T_4* protein binding is normal. Alternatively, your physician can measure the *free T_4* level itself in a sample of your blood, though the latter is a more expensive test.

If more information is needed, your physician will

---

*About 10 percent of the time, your thyroid gland may be making relatively less thyroxine and more of a second thyroid hormone called *triiodothyronine*. If so, a sample of your blood will show a high level of T_3 despite a normal level of T_4. Since *thyrotoxicosis* is another name for hyperthyroidism, this condition has been called *T_3-thyrotoxicosis*.

usually order a *radioactive iodine uptake* test. Determining that your thyroid gland is using a greater-than-normal amount of iodine helps to exclude other causes of hyperthyroidism, such as thyroid inflammation (*thyroiditis*). Often a picture of your thyroid (*thyroid scan*) will be made at the same time in order to find out whether your entire thyroid gland is overactive, as is the case with Graves' disease, or whether just a portion of the gland is hyperfunctioning, as would be the case in a toxic *nodular* goiter (see Chapter 5 and Figure 7 in Chapter 2).

If the diagnosis of hyperthyroidism is still in question, your physician also can perform a test based on the interrelationship between your thyroid gland and the higher brain centers that usually govern its function. As said earlier, your thyroid gland is controlled by your pituitary gland at the base of your brain. The pituitary is, in turn, governed by a higher brain center known as the *hypothalamus* (see Figure 11). Normally, your hypothalamus produces *TSH-releasing hormone (TRH)*, which

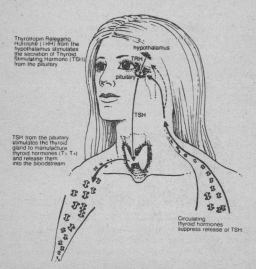

Figure 11   The Hypothalamic-Pituitary-Thyroid Axis.

causes the pituitary to release thyroid stimulating hormone, which in turn stimulates production of T$_3$ and T$_4$ by your thyroid gland. Physicians now use synthetic TRH to test the function of the entire pituitary-thyroid system.

If your pituitary and thyroid glands are healthy, an intravenous injection of TRH stimulates your pituitary to release a certain amount of TSH into your blood stream, where the change in level can easily be checked. In contrast, if you are hyperthyroid, your pituitary TSH-secreting cells have been shut off by the high thyroid hormone levels in your blood, and therefore will not release TSH in response to TRH. Thus, blood tests after an injection of TRH will show no rise in your blood TSH level if you are hyperthyroid. Typical TRH response tests in both normal and hyperthyroid individuals are shown in Figure 12.

Two characteristics of the TRH test have made it extremely popular and most helpful in the diagnosis of

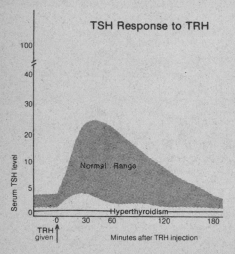

Figure 12   The lower flat line in the graph indicates the lack of TSH response to an injection of TRH in a patient with hyperthyroidism.

hyperthyroidism. First, it is so sensitive that the test can be used to diagnose hyperthyroidism even in its mildest forms. Second, and better still, it does not significantly change your thyroid hormone level. Therefore, it does not worsen the symptoms of hyperthyroidism in hyperthyroid patients.

In past years, if you were young and not very sick, your doctor would try to slow down your thyroid gland by giving you extra thyroid hormone, in the form of tablets containing T3 (Cytomel). In a normal person, the uptake of radioiodine by the thyroid would decrease by more than 50 percent after ten days of the *suppression test*, because the thyroid hormone in the tablets would decrease the pituitary gland's secretion of TSH. This, in turn, would cause a decrease in thyroid function, reflected by a decrease in the thyroid's use of iodine. However, if your thyroid was overactive, it would not be under the control of TSH. Therefore, the uptake would not fall as much (and probably would not fall at all).

Today this suppression test is rarely used, because it can cause problems for you if you are hyperthyroid, for the T3 tablets that you take, plus your own thyroid hormone, may make all of your symptoms worse. As a result, the test can make any hyperthyroid patient sicker and is unnecessarily risky for elderly patients and those with heart disease.

Since the TRH test does not worsen the symptoms of hyperthyroidism, it has replaced the suppression test as an aid in the diagnosis of mild hyperthyroidism. It can be performed in a doctor's office in one hour or less, and results of the test are almost always clear-cut.

Of course, if your routine blood tests are definitely abnormal, the TRH test is unnecessary. Moreover, now there are even new supersensitive *monocolonal antibody* TSH tests, which measure the blood level of TSH much more precisely than ever before. Someday soon these tests may reliably distinguish between hyperthyroidism (TSH low or absent) and normal (TSH normal).

THE TREATMENT OF GRAVES' DISEASE

Rest and sedation were the only treatment available for hyperthyroidism until 1884, when a patient was cured by having part of the thyroid gland removed surgically. In the early days of surgery, however, patients were often so sick with hyperthyroidism that many died during their thyroid operation. It wasn't until the 1920s that we learned to control the severity of hyperthyroidism before the operation by giving patients iodine drops, which slowed down thyroid function. This simple treatment markedly decreased the risk of surgery for patients with Graves' disease. For a while, physicians tried to avoid surgery and treat patients with iodine alone, but although this worked temporarily, control of the disease was unpredictable and many patients suffered a relapse of hyperthyroidism even while continuing to take iodine drops.

Antithyroid drugs,* in use since the early 1940s, represent one of the three major forms of treatment for the hyperthyroidism of Graves' disease that are in current use. These drugs act to prevent the thyroid from manufacturing thyroid hormone. Then, as the production of hormone declines, the symptoms of hyperthyroidism gradually subside. If this is the way your overactive thyroid is treated, you probably will begin to feel better within ten days to two weeks, and you will feel almost well in six to eight weeks.

You will probably take the medication for six to twelve months, after which your physician will probably stop the drug to see if your hyperthyroidism returns. Current studies indicate that you will have about a 30 percent chance of remaining well without medication.

---

*In the United States, propylthiouracil (PTU) and methimazole (Tapazole) are the antithyroid drugs that are used, while British physicians prefer carbimazole, a drug related to methimazole.

You are likely to be one of the fortunate 30 percent if your hyperthyroidism was mild to begin with or if you started treatment within a few months of the beginning of your illness. If you do experience a remission, your family physician will still check you periodically after that to be sure that your thyroid does not become overactive again and also to be sure that thyroid failure does not appear in later years.

Though antithyroid drugs provide an excellent treatment for hyperthyroidism, *they have certain peculiarities that you should know about* if your doctor prescribes them for you. First, because the tablets usually have a short duration of action, your doctor will probably recommend that you take these medications every six to eight hours, at least to begin with. Many people have difficulty remembering the midday doses. Methimazole is preferred by the authors because its longer duration of action allows it to be taken once a day by most patients.

Second, antithyroid drugs cause allergic reactions in about 5 percent of patients who take them. The most common reaction is a skin rash that is usually red and itchy but that, in its extreme form, may have the appearance of generalized hives. Less often, the pills may cause fever, joint pains, or liver disease. A far more serious form of antithyroid drug reaction, which happens to about one of every 300 patients who take the medication, is a decrease in the neutrophil* (white blood cell) count, which may lower your resistance to infections. Therefore, if you are taking one of these drugs and develop a rash, itching, hives, joint pains, or evidence of an infection (such as fever or sore throat), you should stop taking the drug and call your physician *that day*. If your physician determines that your problem is drug allergy, another form of treatment will be recommended. If you have any fever or infection while you are taking an antithyroid medication, you *must* have a white blood cell

---

*In its most extreme form, all the neutrophils may disappear from the blood—a condition known as *agranulocytosis*.

count measured. If the count shows a normal number of neutrophils, your doctor can restart your antithyroid drug even while your infection is being treated. If the neutrophil count is low, your doctor will begin another form of thyroid treatment. Thereafter, your physician will watch you and your blood count very carefully until you are healthy again.

Recent studies suggest the agranulocytosis is more likely to occur in older patients (in whom radioiodine is the preferred treatment anyway) and is more common in patients given propylthiomail than in those given methimazole, as long as the dose of methimazole does not exceed 30 milligrams per day.[5]

Even if your white blood cell count has been lowered by the drug, if these precautions are taken, it will probably return to normal within seven to fourteen days after you stop the medication. But if you continue to take one of these drugs in spite of a falling white blood count, there is risk of a serious and possibly *fatal* outcome. *This possible danger must be thoroughly understood by all who take the drugs*.

If antithyroid drugs have failed to control your hyperthyroidism, or if they are inappropriate for some other reason, doctors can limit your thyroid gland's ability to function with either radioactive iodine or surgery.

Radioactive iodine has been used in the treatment of hyperthyroidism for many years. Studies at the Massachusetts General Hospital that were begun in 1939 demonstrated the treatment's effectiveness, and long-term follow-up studies from many medical centers have confirmed its safety. Radioactive iodine in this treatment is the same isotope (^{131}I) used in many laboratories to test thyroid function in uptake and scan procedures, but the treatment dose is, of course, much larger. Radioiodine is successful in controlling hyperthyroidism because it goes into the thyroid gland and remains there long enough to irradiate—and thus destroy—large amounts of thyroid tissue. Then, within days, it disappears from the body, either eliminated in the urine or transformed by *decay* into a nonradioactive state. If the dosage is calculated correctly, you should be well in three to six months, and that is usually what happens. If you are given too little radioactive iodine, you will remain hyperthyroid, but less so than before. Surprisingly, with so many factors to consider in choosing a proper treatment dose of radioiodine,[6] about 80 percent of patients have their hyperthyroidism controlled with a single treatment. Moreover, those who are still hyperthyroid can be given one or more additional doses of radioiodine until they become well.

You may wonder why every hyperthyroid patient isn't treated this way. Radioactive iodine is tasteless and easily given, usually in a glass of water. It is so readily absorbed that you don't need to be fasting when you are given the treatment. Furthermore, radioactive iodine is usually well-tolerated and painless, though in rare instances patients have complained of a sore throat or mild thyroid tenderness for two or three days.

The greatest concern that we have about radioactive iodine—and the reason that we are particularly reluctant to treat small children in this manner—is concern for possible harm to the thyroid or other parts of the body from the radiation used in the treatment. As outlined in detail in Chapter 12, there is no question that x-rays and other radioactive substances, including radioactive iodine, can cause benign and malignant tumors in human beings who are exposed to large enough quantities of these materials. Yet early worries over possible harmful effects in hyperthyroid patients who were treated with radioiodine have not been borne out in the more than forty years that we have treated patients in this manner. For example, we have not observed any increased risk of leukemia, thyroid cancer, or other tumors in patients treated with radioiodine when compared with similar patients treated with antithyroid drugs or surgery. Additionally, there has been no evidence of infertility or birth defects in children born to women following this treatment. (On the other hand, ^{131}I treatment should *never* be given to a woman *during* pregnancy because of the risk of damage to the thyroid of the unborn child [see Chapter 13]. At present, therefore, our experience leads us to conclude that radioactive iodine is the treatment of choice for hyperthyroidism in most adults. Moreover, it is now being used increasingly in younger patients as well.*

The major problem with radioiodine treatment for *hyper*thyroidism is the subsequent development of *hypo*thyroidism. If you have Graves' disease, your thyroid will probably become underactive at some future time. However, your thyroid will fail sooner after radioiodine than it will after antithyroid drug or surgical treatment of your overactive thyroid. Long-term follow-up studies of patients with Graves' disease who have been treated with radioactive iodine reveal that within ten years up to 90 percent of patients so treated will have become hypothyroid. Nevertheless, late thyroid failure is not necessarily a reason to avoid the use of radioactive iodine to treat this disease, since the immediate necessity is to reduce thyroid hormone production; this is accomplished easily and safely with radioiodine. Furthermore, when the thyroid gland does fail to function, it can be treated safely and easily with hormone tablets taken just once a day.

The key to proper treatment of hyperthyroidism with radioiodine, therefore, is a careful and prolonged follow-up. Unfortunately, a lot of older people were treated with radioiodine many years ago and were told they were "cured" by their radioactive iodine treatment; they were never warned about late thyroid failure because their physicians didn't know it would happen. Therefore, it is our hope that if you have relatives or friends who had radioiodine treatment years ago, you will urge them to

---

*See Chapter 11 for a discussion of the risk and merits of this treatment in children for whom there are additional important considerations.

see their physician for a follow-up thyroid evaluation.

If your physician decides to treat your thyroid with radioactive iodine, it will be because the expected benefits from the treatment outweigh the small risk of harmful side effects from the radioiodine to your thyroid and the rest of your body. But when you return home after your treatment, the radioactive iodine in your body can affect those around you. Although the risk to them from your radioiodine is small, if you take some simple precautions you can minimize their exposure to your radioactivity.

Most of the radioactivity will be eliminated from your body in your urine within 48 hours, so those two days are the important time for precautions. During that time, your radioactivity can affect those around you, their exposure depending upon *how long they are with you* and *how far away they are from you*. Thus, we advise our patients to minimize the time they are in close contact with others. Since infants and small children are the most sensitive to such radiation, make a special point of avoiding prolonged close contact with them. For example, let someone else hold and feed babies while you sit farther away.*

Since radioactive iodine is present in the urine, elderly patients who have problems with bladder control must be especially careful in using the bathroom during the first two days after such treatment. Since the radioiodine will also be in saliva, we advise our patients to avoid kissing anyone for 48 hours. Finally, radioiodine will be present in breast milk, so if you are breastfeeding you will have to stop nursing until your doctor says it is safe to start again.

When actual measurements have been carried out in patients' homes, it has been found that very little radiation is given to family members by a treated patient. Nevertheless, these simple precautions are worth taking to keep that exposure to a minimum. The U.S. Nuclear

*Since the radiation effect you have upon those around you falls off as the *square* of the distance between you, you will have a negligible effect on anyone more than three feet away.

Regulatory Commission is currently preparing a pamphlet for patients treated with radioiodine that will provide general information about radiation safety in a more comprehensive manner.

Your hyperthyroidism can also be cured by means of *surgery* in which most of your thyroid gland is removed. Following such a procedure, the thyroid tissue that remains in your neck still may be hyperactive; but since the amount of tissue is less, it cannot produce as much thyroid hormone. Thus, your thyroid hormone blood levels will fall and your symptoms of hyperthyroidism will subside.

To prepare you for surgery, your physician probably will control your thyroid function by treating you for a few weeks with an antithyroid drug. Iodine drops are also usually prescribed during the ten days just before surgery so that there will be less bleeding during your operation.

Most surgeons remove about 90 percent of the thyroid gland in order to be sure that enough tissue is removed to cure the patient. Hypothyroidism may occur immediately after surgery, or may develop later, but if it does occur, it can be treated easily with thyroid hormone tablets. Patients taking thyroid tablets should feel completely well if their dose of thyroid hormone is correct.

If you elect to have surgical treatment, the major concern for you and your doctor should be the choice of the surgeon who will perform your operation. Head and neck surgery requires the skills of an expert, and most large hospitals have certain surgeons who perform most of the thyroid surgery. The choice of the surgeon is important because surgical complications may be serious. The *recurrent laryngeal nerves*, which supply your vocal cords, pass very near to the thyroid (Figure 13). If your surgeon accidentally cuts one of these nerves during the operation, you will be immediately and permanently hoarse. There is also danger of damage to the parathy-

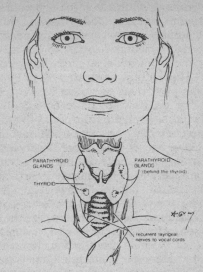

PARATHYROID
GLANDS

PARATHYROID
GLANDS
(behind the thyroid)

THYROID

recurrent laryngeal
nerves to vocal cords

Figure 18   A hypothyroid patient responds to an injection
of TRH by producing excessive amounts of TSH.

roid glands, which control your blood calcium level. If
that occurs, you may need medication the rest of your
life. Many patients want to know what sort of scar to
expect after a thyroid operation. Actually, most are almost invisible within several months.

In summary, if a skilled, experienced thyroid surgeon
is not available, radioactive iodine or antithyroid drugs
are safer forms of therapy for the hyperthyroidism of
Graves' disease. On the other hand, if you are allergic to
antithyroid drugs or do not want to take radioactive iodine, thyroid surgery can be a very good way to control
an overactive thyroid.

No matter which of the three main methods of treatment
you and your physician decide upon, your doctor may
also prescribe a *beta adrenergic blocking drug*, such as

atenolol or *propanolol*, to block the action of circulating thyroid hormone on your body tissues, slowing your heart rate, lessening nervousness, and generally improving your symptoms within minutes to hours, depending on whether the medication is given by injection or in tablet form. These drugs work so well in hyperthyroidism that some physicians use them as the sole form of therapy for the disease, but more commonly, they are given for temporary relief until thyroid function can be controlled permanently by a more traditional method.

Beta-blocking agents have some disadvantages for a few patients: they may make asthma worse and may decrease the strength of heart muscle contraction in patients with heart failure. However, since more hyperthyroid patients are young, the latter complication is rarely encountered. Lesser concerns are the drugs' duration of action, which sometimes makes it necessary for patients to take the pills three or four times a day. The authors prefer atenolol (Tenormin) and related long-acting drugs of this type to the shorter-acting "parent drug" propanolol (Inderal) because of the more convenient once-a-day dosage. Diabetics should know that these drugs may obscure the warning signs of low blood sugar (hypoglycemia). Finally, because they can inhibit the growth of an unborn child and interfere with the breathing of a newborn baby, beta-blocking agents are not recommended for long-term use in pregnancy or for use near the time of delivery if another treatment is available.[7] In spite of all these potential problems, these drugs are usually so safe they are now in common use in the early stages of treatment of many hyperthyroid patients. They make them feel better until their thyroid glands can be controlled by other means.

Another form of therapy is *iodine*. Although iodine alone is not a good treatment for hyperthyroidism, it is often used in conjunction with surgery (noted above) or after radioactive iodine treatment. During the three to six months while you wait for the radioactive iodine to work, your doctor may prescribe iodine drops, which may control the hyperthyroidism temporarily. These drugs will be withdrawn gradually as your hyperthyroidism subsides from the radioactive iodine treatment.

New drugs are constantly under investigation because every treatment has some possible complications. Most patients, however, are easily and safely managed by one of the standard time-tested remedies: antithyroid drugs, radioiodine, or a thyroid operation. But no matter what the therapeutic approach, *every patient treated for hyperthyroidism must have at least an annual follow-up examination, including measurements of serum T_4 and TSH concentrations, for the rest of his or her life*. In this way when hypothyroidism does develop it will be promptly detected and treated. In summary, if you have Graves' disease, your overactive thyroid will probably slow down someday and become underactive. This will happen earlier if the treatment used to control your hyperthyroidism is radioiodine or surgery (both of which damage your thyroid) than if your treatment is with antithyroid drugs alone. It would probably happen, though perhaps not for many years, if you are not treated at all.[8] In short, the natural history of Graves' disease appears to be a slow but progressive decline in thyroid function in later years that can be hastened by antithyroid treatment that damages your thyroid gland.[9]

GRAVES' DISEASE

BY L. H.

I am 27 years old, and I have had Graves' disease for the past year. In June of 1973 I started having vague symptoms that my husband and I overlooked as normal. The only problem that bothered me was the constant sensation of having sand in my eyes. Then, practically overnight, they became inflamed, swollen, and itchy. I immediately went to an eye doctor who diagnosed a viral infection. But, during the rest of the summer my eyes continued to fluctuate between being normal or being symptomatic. I never once thought the other things that were happening to me could be related, and so I never mentioned them to the eye doctor who saw me.

I have always been extremely conscious of my weight, and so when I found that I had lost 15 pounds over the course of the summer, I thought it was so terrific I didn't even question it. I suddenly could eat anything I wanted, in any quantity, and I wouldn't gain any weight.

I work on a ward in a hospital and it is not air conditioned. Thus, any intolerance to heat seemed natural. Everyone complained of the heat, but I seemed to feel it more and to sweat more than anyone else.

Weight loss and heat intolerance were the only two symptoms I had during the first few months of my disease. At the end of the summer, however, everything seemed to reach a peak almost overnight. I knew something was very wrong when my eyes became prominent and my lids retracted to the point where I could not close my eyes easily. I couldn't sleep well at night. I was very jumpy and irritable with people around me. After doing the mildest form of exercise my legs would feel like rubber and start shaking. I kept having bouts of diarrhea, and my heart felt it was pounding very hard.

My overactive thyroid was discovered by my doctor at the end of the summer and suddenly all of these symptoms made sense. I wasn't sick because my husband or anyone else was trying to provoke me and irritate me; it was me all along. Unfortunately, my being so jumpy and excitable at this time made it very hard for me to accept my disease. I felt as if I was constantly wound up and the slightest provocation would cause me to explode. It's a terrible feeling to know that you are hurting people around you and that you can't control yourself. It was finally necessary for me to leave work. The heat and frustration of my job were just too much for me to cope with.

My husband and I wanted very much to start a family about the time my illness began, but when I was started on Tapazole, an antithyroid drug, I was advised not to become pregnant while on this drug. This, too, made it very difficult for me to accept my disease, but I had decided on surgery as my course of treatment and felt that, hopefully, all would be cured in a few months.

I was told that with a thyroidectomy as my plan of treatment, I would have to be on Tapazole for only six to eight weeks, at which time my thyroid level would be low enough so that I could have my thyroid removed. But it was very difficult for me to keep busy and try to ignore all that was suddenly happening to my body. I was home alone all day and really could do nothing except feel very sorry for myself. I wanted so much to become pregnant, but I was bothered even more by my change in appearance. My eyes, I felt, had altered my looks considerably and I was embarrassed and ashamed to go out in public. It is pretty difficult to hide a drastic change or disfigurement on one's face, and the constant stares and questions were problems with which I was unable to cope.

I was sent to an eye doctor who taught me how to tape my eyes shut at night. If I did not tape them, they did not quite close while I slept, which was the cause for much of their irritation. Gradually, my eyes started to feel a lot better and the emotional impact of having to tape them subsided.

I had my surgery in January and all went well. I honestly don't remember any discomfort, except for a stiff neck. The problem that occurred was with my eyes. It was necessary for me to go to the Massachusetts Eye and Ear Infirmary for five days because of an ulcer on my cornea. This was taken care of, but I had to take cortisone pills for a month and a half to reduce the inflammation of my eyes. I was frightened over the prospect of having to stay on this medication for a long time. My vision remained blurred for a good six weeks after surgery and this compounded my fear. The realization that I might have serious eye problems for the rest of my life was truly frightening.

It is now a year since I first became sick. My eyes have improved considerably since the time of surgery. It is still necessary to tape them at night, but my eye doctor does not think I'll have to do this for more than another few months. I feel a lot better than I did a year ago, but things have yet to be resolved. I am on thyroid pills, probably for the rest of my life, and it is not certain what dosage I will have to take. It will take a few months for my body to stabilize and a permanent dosage to be determined.

After working in a hospital and seeing so many horrible diseases, my first reaction to discovering I had Graves' disease was rather mild. I was thankful that it wasn't anything truly serious. I am still thankful, but also aware that hyperthyroidism can be serious if not treated properly. The treatment of my Graves' disease took a long time and it was very frustrating. But I am sure now that with the steady improvement of my eyes and the stabilization of my body, I will soon feel like the "true me" again.

It is now five years since I became ill and so many things have occurred since I last wrote this account that I must update it.

I am still taking thyroid pills daily, but the dosage has basically been the same for years. I have my blood drawn about once a year to determine whether my dosage is too high or low. I am now so aware of what is normal that I can usually decide if my medication is correct or not.

I no longer have to tape my eyes at night, but still use an ointment to keep them lubricated and protected in case I should open them while sleeping. I feel that I will never really look the same as I did before I developed Graves' disease, but I definitely feel that I've improved tremendously since I first got sick. When I meet new people, I no longer feel self-conscious or obligated to give an explanation about my appearance. Whenever I tell new friends about my experience they are genuinely surprised and tell me they never noticed anything wrong with my eyes.

The most important thing to bring up to date about myself, however, is the fact that I have had two beautiful and healthy children since I last updated my story. I became pregnant with my son seven months after my surgery, and he is now four years old. I also have a seven-week-old daughter, and needless to say, my husband and I are thrilled with our family. Both my pregnancies and deliveries were normal and had absolutely no complications. I had some difficulty conceiving my first child, but I honestly feel that it was because it was so soon after my thyroid surgery. I was followed very closely during both pregnancies to make sure my medication dosages were correct and my thyroid level was normal. Both children are normal and healthy and a great joy to us.

When I reread this account or think back on when I first became ill it seems so long ago and vague now. I have gone through many changes, but I feel I've been very fortunate. My eyes and body have stabilized, and I finally feel like the "true me" again.

HYPERTHYROIDISM TREATED BY RADIOACTIVE IODINE

by R. D'A.

Because I had had a hysterectomy in April 1977 at age forty-nine, all my symptoms were attributed to the menopause. The subtle happenings to my system seemed natural after major surgery of this type. My pulse raced at the least exertion, and at times I had palpitations even while sitting still. I was extremely nervous and the heat of the summer seemed more intense than in other summers. My body was always moist and clammy. Thinking this was so-called "hot flashes," I tried to ignore the condition as best I could. The muscles in my arms and legs were so weak that I even had trouble opening a jar or getting out of a chair. Even climbing stairs made my legs feel tired.

As the summer moved along, other changes began to annoy me: itching eyes, shaky hands, fingernails that were wrinkled and hard to keep clean, and a steady loss of weight. I told myself it was all nerves from the sudden onset of menopause.

Finally, I was hospitalized in August because of exhaustion. The nurse who admitted me said my pulse rate was 140 per minute. The doctor said she suspected a thyroid condition and ordered blood tests and a thyroid scan. The test results confirmed her suspicion: hyperthyroidism.

The doctor began to give me propylthiouracil pills to treat my condition. I was told that "PTU" (I could never remember the whole name) would slow down my thyroid and make me feel better. Sure enough, in about a week I began to feel calmer and my pulse began to slow down. By the end of a month I was almost back to normal—sweating less, no palpitations, and even a little stronger. Also, I began to gain back some of the 15 pounds of weight I had lost over the summer.

My doctor explained that although PTU was helping me feel better, it was likely that if I stopped the medication my thyroid condition would probably come right back. Therefore in November I was referred to a thyroid specialist for further treatment.

For a while this new doctor had me continue the PTU, until blood tests confirmed that my thyroid level was indeed normal. He explained that because my thyroid had been overactive for a long time, and because it had not gotten smaller while I took PTU, that PTU probably would not cure my condition. The doctor said that he didn't like to use PTU for treatment for very long in someone who wasn't likely to be cured by it, because sometimes it hurt the white blood cells and might lead to an infection or other serious complications. He said that if I got an infection or fever while taking PTU, I should have a white cell count taken at my local hospital and not to start PTU again until I got a report from him. Fortunately this was never necessary.

He discussed with me the other ways my thyroid condition could be treated: surgery or "RAI" (radioactive iodine). Both treatments were fully explained. His recommendation in my particular case was RAI. I was assured of the safety of RAI, and since I had full confidence in his choice of treatment, I agreed. In December PTU was stopped for 3 days and a radioactive iodine uptake test was taken. The result was shown to me and thoroughly explained. Later that morning, the doctor administered the RAI "drink," which was in a small paper cup. It was tasteless, colorless, odorless, and—best of all—painless. The most difficult part of taking the RAI was the fact that I knew it was a radioactive chemical. It was over in a few seconds and I was on my way home.

One week later, I resumed taking PTU while I waited for the radioiodine to have a chance to work completely. Ultimately I stopped the PTU in March of 1978 and have remained completely well since then. A follow-up thyroid check once a year is all that is necessary. I do not take medication of any kind. I am now feeling great and I'm very thankful.

I have been told that my thyroid may gradually slow down sometime in the coming years, and that is the reason for my yearly "checkups." I also know that if my thyroid does slow down, I can take a thyroid pill once a day to make up the difference and keep my body healthy.

CHAPTER FIVE

The Overactive Thyroid

Other Forms of Hyperthyroidism

In the preceding chapter, we described a form of hyperthyroidism known as Grave's disease in which your entire thyroid gland becomes overactive. The term *hyperthyroidism* also includes several other disorders in which a greater-than-normal amount of thyroid hormone circulates in your blood stream, with the result that you may feel sick in much the same way as you would if you had Grave's disease. You may get nervous and feel jumpy, dislike hot weather, and prefer cool temperatures, and you may experience attacks of rapid heart palpitations. In addition, you may lose weight even though you seem to eat a normal or greater-than-normal amount of food.

The kinds of hyperthyroidism described in this chapter differ from Graves' disease in several important ways:

—Graves' disease seems to occur in individuals who have inherited a tendency or susceptibility to that condition, which is then triggered by some additional factor (such as a stressful life situation). There does not appear to be as much of an inherited tendency in these other forms of hyperthyroidism.

—For Graves' disease, there is good evidence that a gradual slowing of thyroid function is part of the natural course of the disease in its late stages. Lifelong follow-up is important, to recognize and treat hypothyroidism when it occurs. These other kinds of hyperthyroidism do not show this tendency to subsequent thyroid gland failure. Instead, many of these disorders go away by themselves or can be cured completely by appropriate treatment.

—Graves' disease begins most often in women between the ages of 20 and 40. Though most of these other types of hyperthyroidism are also more common in women than men, they tend to affect people of different ages. *Toxic multinodular goiter*, for example, most commonly begins between the ages of 30 and 50.

—Patients with Graves' disease have a tendency toward developing certain other apparently related conditions. These include protrusion of the eyes (exophthalmos), lumpy skin over the shins (pretibial myxedema), and other associated autoimmune conditions (see Chapter 9). There do not seem to be similar tendencies in patients who have other forms of hyperthyroidism.

—In Graves' disease, substances known as *antibodies* appear in the blood and cause the thyroid to become overactive. These *thyroid stimulating antibodies* do not appear to play a role in causing other forms of hyperthyroidism.

—Finally, these other kinds of hyperthyroidism are less common than Graves' disease.

With these differences in mind, we will proceed to a discussion of the important features of these other diseases that can produce hyperthyroidism.

THE HOT NODULE

Overactivity of a single thyroid nodule, actually a type of harmless thyroid tumor, accounts for about 5 percent of all hyperthyroidism. It is sometimes called a "hot nodule" because of its appearance in a thyroid scan, (Figure 14) but may also be referred to as *Plummer's disease* in honor of the Mayo Clinic physician who first described hyperthyroidism due to overactive nodules in 1913. Single overactive thyroid nodules are usually discovered in older women, but may occur at any age and in either sex.

If you have diffuse toxic goiter (Graves' disease) your entire thyroid gland produces excessive amounts of thyroid hormones. If you have a hot nodule, however, only that nodule in your thyroid is functioning excessively. Gradually, as the nodule produces more and more hormone, the rest of your gland decreases its function. Finally a time is reached at which the nodule makes enough thyroid hormone to meet the needs of your whole body. But as long as the total amount of hormone made by the nodule is still "normal" for your body, you won't feel sick. It is only when the nodule makes *more* than enough hormone that you begin to notice symptoms of hyperthyroidism.

Sometimes, a physician examining you can suspect a "hot nodule" as the cause of your hyperthyroid condition even before tests are performed. The clues to the diagnosis are:

—You are hyperthyroid.

—Only one lump is enlarged in your thyroid, rather than the entire gland.

—The rest of your thyroid gland may feel smaller than normal, since it has stopped working because your nodule is making more than enough thyroid hormone for your whole body.

—Unlike a patient with Graves' disease, who often has relatives who have had a thyroid problem or other "related" conditions (see Chapter 8), if you have a hot nodule you are less likely to have a "positive" family history.

It is usually an easy matter for your doctor to prove that your hyperthyroidism is due to a hot nodule. A sample of your blood will contain a high level of thyroid hormone (either T_3 alone or both T_3 and T_4), and your thyroid scan will show a single active area of function corresponding to your nodule (Figure 14).

We don't know what causes part of your thyroid gland to become overactive in this manner, so we don't know how to keep it from happening to you. Fortunately, most patients with a hot nodule do not seem to become quite as sick as most of those who have Graves' disease. If your hot nodule does not produce hyperthyroidism,

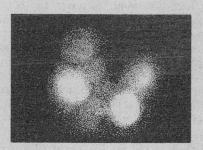

Figure 14 An artist's rendering of a thyroid scan shows that all of the radioiodine has been concentrated in an overactive nodule, which is making so much thyroid hormone that the rest of the thyroid is inactive.

your physician may simply examine you at periodic intervals, checking your thyroid hormone blood levels.

In contrast to Graves' disease, antithyroid drug treatment will not lead to a remission (cure) of this form of hyperthyroidism. Therefore these drugs are rarely used to treat hot nodules. If your nodule produces so much hormone that it makes you ill, your physician may advise that it be removed in an operation. Surgery should cure you, since only the nodule need be removed, and the rest of your thyroid gland can be left alone. Your normal thyroid tissue will start functioning again once the nodule has been removed, making hypothyroidism after surgery a rare occurrence.

Alternatively, your physician may recommend treatment of your hot nodule with *radioactive iodine*. Radioactive iodine, usually swallowed in a drink of water, goes to your thyroid, where it is collected only by the hot nodule, since the rest of the thyroid is inactive. It remains in the nodule for several days until it is either eliminated from your body in your urine or is transformed to a nonradioactive state by a process known as *decay*. However, during its short stay in your thyroid nodule, it destroys some of your thyroid tissue. If enough tissue is destroyed or damaged in such a way that it can no longer make thyroid hormone, you will be cured. For reasons we do not understand, such nodules usually require a larger dose of radioiodine than is needed to cure patients with Graves' disease. But in spite of the larger dose of radioactive iodine required, hypothyroidism rarely follows such treatment, since the rest of the thyroid largely escapes radiation damage.* Weeks later, when your hot nodule slows its function as a result of radiation effect, the rest of your thyroid gland

*As indicated in several different parts of this book—most notably Chapter 11—physicians are concerned about possible serious consequences to your body any time we use radioactive materials. To date there is no evidence that this treatment has caused thyroid tumors or other forms of cancer in adults, and the authors believe that the benefits of radioiodine outweigh its theoretical risks.

will start working again. You should then feel well and be permanently cured.

TOXIC MULTINODULAR GOITER

Sometimes there are several overactive nodules in your thyroid, and this is another form of Plummer's disease. This condition, known as *toxic multinodular goiter*, causes about 25 percent of all hyperthyroidism and is about half as common as Graves' disease. Patients tend to be older than those who get Graves' disease, and therefore they may get sicker from the rapid pulse, weakness, and weight loss that occur because of the high level off thyroid hormone. In most cases, a goiter has been present for many years, gradually becoming more and more overactive until hyperthyroidism develops.

If you have a toxic multinodular goiter, your physician may suspect this condition because you will have symptoms of hyperthyroidism and an enlarged, lumpy-feeling thyroid gland. The diagnosis is usually confirmed by a blood test that shows a high level of thyroid hormone and by a thyroid scan that demonstrates several areas of increased thyroid activity (Figure 15).

Since we don't know what causes a nodular goiter to become hyperactive, we cannot prevent the onset of this condition, but treatment of this form of hyperthyroidism is usually straightforward. If you are sick because of the high level of thyroid hormone in your system when you first see your physician, your symptoms can be helped promptly with a *beta adrenergic blocking drug*, such as atenolol or propanolol, which blocks the action of the hormone on your body, slowing your pulse and generally making you feel better. In addition, an antithyroid drug such as propylthiouracil or methimazole (Tapazole) can be used to slow down production of hormone by the overactive thyroid nodules. But since toxic multinodular goiter does not tend to subside by itself (as sometimes

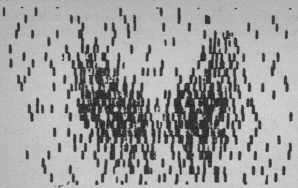

Figure 15 An artist's rendering of the thyroid scan of a patient with a toxic multinodular goiter shows several areas of increased activity.

occurs in Graves' disease), permanent control of the condition is unlikely unless your physician decreases the number of overactive cells in your thyroid gland.

This may be accomplished by radioactive iodine treatment, but the effects of treatment are slightly different from those encountered with a hot nodule. Since the radioiodine goes into several overactive parts of your thyroid, it is more likely that you will become hypothyroid sometime in the future. Similarly, if thyroid surgery is chosen for a toxic multinodular goiter, the surgeon will probably cure such a patient only if *most* of the thyroid gland is removed during the operation, making hypothyroidism after surgery more likely. If too much tissue is left behind, hyperthyroidism may recur, since new nodules may develop and produce excessive amounts of the hormone.

By either method, the hyperthyroidism can be safely controlled, and if hypothyroidism results from the treatment, it is a simple matter to raise your thyroid hormone blood level to normal with thyroid hormone tablets taken once a day. Your physician will probably want to test your thyroid periodically in the years that follow, since overactive nodules may reappear and change the level of thyroid hormone in your system, possibly even causing hyperthyroidism again. If that happens, the principles of treatment will be the same as before, and usually will involve the use of more radioactive iodine or a second thyroid operation.

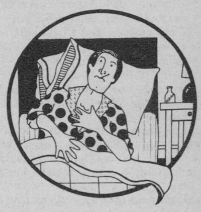

Figure 16 A patient with subacute thyroiditis feels sick and has a tender, inflamed thyroid.

HYPERTHYROIDISM ASSOCIATED WITH THYROID INFLAMMATION

Sometimes, in association with a viral infection, a form of thyroid inflammation known as *subacute thyroiditis* develops. If you have subacute thyroiditis, you may think you have the flu or a very bad sore throat, for you will probably have fever, ache all over, and have a very sore neck because of your tender, inflamed thyroid gland (Figure 16). Thyroid hormone tends to leak out of the inflamed gland, and if enough gets into your system, symptoms of hyperthyroidism may appear. Since your thyroid is not overactive, your doctor can identify this form of hyperthyroidism because you will have an elevated blood level of thyroid hormone, yet a low radioiodine uptake (proof of the gland's inactivity). A high *red blood cell sedimentation rate* is another essential factor helping your doctor make this diagnosis, for it reflects the degree of thyroid inflammation. Since the disease is self-limited, treatment with aspirin for your sore neck, fever, and aching muscles, and a beta adrenergic blocking drug like atenolol or propranolol for your symptoms of hyperthyroidism are usually sufficient. Prompt improvement can be expected and complete cure should follow within two to three months. Very rarely, a period of hypothyroidism can follow the hyperthyroid phase of this illness. This usually is mild, lasts no more than a month, and represents the time it takes for your thyroid to start working again. If you feel sluggish and tired because of the low thyroid hormone level, your physician may prescribe thyroid hormone tablets, but usually this is not necessary.

Spontaneously resolving hyperthyroidism is a condition that has only recently been recognized. It shares many of the features of hyperthyroidism associated with subacute thyroiditis: Patients have high blood levels of thyroid hormones but a low radioiodine uptake. Unlike most patients with subacute thyroiditis, however, patients with this condition do not have a painful thyroid gland or a very high red blood cell sedimentation rate. In short, they lack the symptoms and signs of thyroid inflammation. Furthermore, the disease can recur in the same patient several times, and seems to appear more often after pregnancy. Neither of these features is seen in typical subacute thyroiditis.

If you develop this condition you will be treated as if you had subacute thyroiditis, except that you won't need aspirin since the disease is not painful. Usually, your physician will control your hyperthyroid symptoms with a drug like atenolol or propranolol until the disease subsides spontaneously in a few weeks. A period of hypothyroidism can follow the hyperthyroidism, similar to that seen in subacute thyroiditis. Treatment is rarely required in this circumstance. Recent studies suggest that this form of hyperthyroidism may be associated with thyroid failure later in life, so periodic checkups are important if you have had spontaneously resolving hyperthyroidism.

HYPERTHYROIDISM CAUSED BY IODINE

It has been known for many years that iodine can cause hyperthyroidism in certain susceptible individuals, but the reasons for this curious phenomenon are unknown. Before 1972, the problem was seen only in iodine-deficient areas of the world. When needed dietary iodine supplements were introduced into the food in those areas, some of the inhabitants developed hyperthyroidism. Sometimes the hyperthyroidism went away by itself, but usually it had to be controlled by drugs, radioactive iodine, or thyroid surgery.

More recently, we have learned that excessive iodine may cause hyperthyroidism even in individuals who have normal amounts of iodine in their diets. Excessive iodine might come from iodine in foods such as kelp (seaweed), in medications such as expectorants, or in x-ray dyes such as those used to x-ray the kidneys, gall bladder, spinal canal, or blood vessels. Patients with underlying nodular goiters are the ones most likely to experience this "thyrotoxic" effect of iodine.

If you have hyperthyroidism due to excessive iodine, your physician will first try to see that your extra iodine intake is stopped. Second, your symptoms will probably be controlled with atenolol, propranolol, or one of the other beta adrenergic blocking drugs until it is determined whether your thyroid overactivity will subside spontaneously. If you remain hyperthyroid, other measures can be taken. Your treatment may include antithyroid drugs as well as surgical removal of the thyroid gland. Radioactive iodine treatment is not successful in the early stages of this condition because the excess iodine already present in your system dilutes the therapeutic effect of the radioactive iodine.*

OVERMEDICATION WITH THYROID HORMONE

Hyperthyroidism may occur in anyone who is taking too much thyroid hormone. Emotionally disturbed patients have been known to take too much hormone intentionally; they are best advised to seek help for their problem rather than hurt themselves with medicine. On the other hand, this kind of problem is sometimes observed in individuals who have no intention of causing themselves trouble. It may seem simple and obvious that you should not take too much thyroid hormone or the wrong kind of thyroid hormone, but we are now learning that it is not always so simple. Medical studies show that if your own thyroid gland is underactive, you probably require a daily dose of no more than 150 to 200 micrograms of thyroxine* (equal to one and one half to two grains of desiccated thyroid)* as adequate replacement therapy.

*See Chapter 14 for a full discussion of the possible dangers that can be caused by either too much or too little iodine.
*According to chemical tests, in America the most reliably potent preparations of thyroxine are Levothroid and Synthroid. In Canada, there is Eltroxin in addition to Synthroid. Generic substitutes are not reliably potent and therefore cannot be recommended.
*If you are currently taking desiccated thyroid tablets there is good reason to talk with your physician about changing to thyroxine. A full discussion of the reasons for which is advisable can be found in Chapter 6.

If you are taking more than this amount of thyroxine, you may have symptoms of hyperthyroidism *due to the medication itself.* Your physician can perform tests that will tell accurately whether your thyroid hormone dosage is correct or excessive, so if you are concerned about your treatment you should review your dosage with your physician. If there is a question of hyperthyroidism, your dosage can be gradually reduced until a rise in your blood level of thyroid stimulating hormone (TSH) signals that your pituitary gland senses too little thyroid in your system. At that point, your physician can increase your dosage slightly to normalize your serum TSH. Once your thyroid hormone needs are known, your physician probably will not need to check your thyroid hormone and TSH levels more than once a year.

TUMORS THAT CAN CAUSE HYPERTHYROIDISM

Several kinds of tumors have been found to be an occasional cause of hyperthyroidism. Thyroid cancer is one such tumor. Sometimes thyroid cancer cells are able to make thyroid hormone, and when there are enough cells present in your body, hyperthyroidism may occur.

Very rarely, tumors in other parts of the body can influence your thyroid. For example, there are a few reports of patients in whom pituitary gland tumors have made excessive amounts of TSH. Here, treatment is usually best directed against the pituitary (which is the real culprit), rather than against the thyroid, which, in this instance, is an innocent bystander. Other rare tumors that have caused hyperthyroidism have occurred in the reproductive system. When they are recognized they are dealt with directly through treatment aimed at the source of the problem.

CHAPTER SIX

The Underactive Thyroid

Hypothyroidism and Myxedema

Mrs. S., aged 46, was shown at a meeting of the Northumberland and Durham Medical Society on February 12th, 1881 ... At the time of this meeting she presented the typical features of an advanced case of myxedema ... The experimental nature of the treatment was explained, and the patient, realizing the otherwise hopeless outlook, promptly consented to this trial ... The thyroid gland was removed from a freshly killed sheep with sterilized instruments and conveyed at once in a sterilized bottle to the laboratory where the glycerine extract was prepared ... In the treatment of this case, a hypodermic injection of 25 minims of extract was given twice a week at first, and later on at longer intervals. The patient steadily improved, and three months later ... the condition was thus described:

"The swelling has gradually diminished ... and the face ... has greatly improved in appearance and has much more expression, as many of the natural wrinkles have returned. The speech has become more rapid and fluent ... she answers questions much more readily, the mind has become more active, and the memory has improved. She is more active in all her movements and finds that it requires much less effort than formerly to do her housework ... the skin has been much less dry and she perspires when walking ... she is no longer sensitive to cold ..."

After this, the injections were given at fortnightly intervals, and later on ... she took 10 minims by mouth six nights a week. The patient was then enabled to live in good health for over twenty-eight years after she had reached an advanced stage of myxedema. During this period she consumed over nine pints of liquid thyroid extract or its equivalent, prepared from the thyroid glands of more than 870 sheep.

> —From the "Life-history of the first case of myxedema treated by thyroid extract" by George R. Murray, M.D. The patient was treated from 1891 until her death in 1919. (*British Medical Journal* 1 [1920]: 359.)

When the thyroid gland fails to produce a normal amount of thyroid hormone, a condition known as *hypothyroidism* results. In a survey done many years ago at several large hospitals, less than one patient in a thousand was reported as having hypothyroidism, so it was assumed to be a relatively uncommon disorder. In recent years, however, improved methods for identifying mild degrees of thyroid failure have revealed that the true prevalence of hypothyroidism in the population is much higher. Of even greater interest was a recent survey that found elevated blood levels of *thyroid stimulating hormone* (TSH) in 75 of every thousand women (7.5 percent) and 28 of every thousand men tested.[10] Most physicians believe that elevated TSH levels represent the earliest sign of thyroid failure, and that many such patients will go on to develop more evidence of hypothyroidism.

Thyroid hormones act upon *receptors* in tissues throughout your body. Therefore, it is not surprising that the complaints that you develop in hypothyroidism may involve many different parts of your system. Thyroid hormones control the *rate* at which various things happen, such as the speed of chemical reactions, the rate of tissue growth, and the rate at which electrical impulses travel in your nerves and muscles. So when you become hypothyroid, many of the affected bodily functions simply slow down.

As your thyroid begins to fail, you may *feel* perfectly well, for often the only suggestion of a problem will be a slight enlargement of your thyroid gland (goiter), appearing as a lump in front of your neck. Then, as your thyroid hormone level falls further, you may begin to feel tired and listless, perhaps chilly when those about you are uncomfortably warm. As your skin, hair, and fingernails grow more slowly, they become thickened, dry, and brittle. Some hair loss may be noticed. Then, as your hypothyroidism becomes more severe, changes may occur in the tissues beneath your skin that lead to a characteristic puffy, swollen appearance known as *myxedema*. This is often particularly apparent around your face and eyes.

Your circulation is affected and your heart rate slows, but you probably won't notice this unless someone happens to count your pulse (it may be below 60 beats per minute). Since your intestinal activity slows down, you may become constipated. A few pounds of weight gain may occur due to water retention, but you are not likely to get fat due to hypothyroidism alone. Your muscles may become sore and you may be awakened at night with leg cramps. Muscle swelling may occur and may make your tongue (which is a muscle) bigger. Your nervous system may be affected in several ways. You may notice some memory loss, and you may become more sensitive to medications, so that weak sedatives cause prolonged sleep. Some patients experience tingling in their fingers, or loss of balance and difficulty in walking.

If you are a younger woman, changes in your reproductive system may cause longer, heavier, and more frequent menstruation. Your ovaries may stop producing an egg each month, and, if so, it may be difficult for you to get pregnant. If pregnancy does occur, you are a little more likely to have a miscarriage than if you had a healthy thyroid.

In summary, if you become hypothyroid, the *most* common complaints you are likely to have are feeling "rundown" and "slowed-up." However, subtle changes are probably occurring all over your body as a result of your low thyroid hormone levels.

WHAT CAUSES HYPOTHYROIDISM?

The causes of hypothyroidism vary somewhat with the age of that the disorder begins. Most children born with severe hypothyroidism (cretinism) have never developed enough thyroid tissue to supply adequate amounts of thyroid hormones for their bodily needs. Other hypothyroid infants may have an inherited defect in the production of thyroid hormones within their thyroid gland. In some underdeveloped countries, dietary iodine deficiency is an important added cause of serious hypothyroidism in newborn babies. Although iodine deficiency is no longer a problem in the United States, the opposite condition—iodine excess in pregnancy—still does occur. If a woman consumes too much iodine (usually in medication) during pregnancy, the result may be that her unborn baby's thyroid slows its production of thyroid hormone in the presence of the extra iodine. If so, her baby may be born with hypothyroidism and a goiter.

In older children and adults, a silent, ongoing inflammation (without evidence of infection) of the thyroid, known as *chronic lymphocytic thyroiditis* (also known as *Hashimoto's disease*, in honor of the Japanese physician who described it), is the most common cause of thyroid gland failure. The thyroid fails because inflammation and scarring damage the thyroid tissue. At some point, enough tissue will have been destroyed so that which remains can no longer produce an adequate amount of thyroid hormone to meet the body's needs. (See Chapter 7 for a more complete discussion of thyroiditis.)

Thyroid failure is also very common among patients who have been treated in the past for an overactive thyroid. Here, hypothyroidism may occur immediately after a treatment that destroys or removes part of the thyroid (radioactive iodine or an operation), but, in most instances, the thyroid doesn't fail until months or years later. Such a delayed onset of hypothyroidism suggests that the original treatment is not the only cause of thyroid failure in such patients. Coexistent chronic lymphocytic thyroiditis may be a factor as well.

Less commonly, the thyroid may fail temporarily after a viral infection (see subacute thyroiditis, Chapter 7) or because of a medication. For example, if an antithyroid drug used to control an overactive thyroid is given in too large a dose, hypothyroidism may result and last until the dosage of that drug is reduced. Lithium, a psychiatric drug, can also cause hypothyroidism in some people. Furthermore, some individuals have thyroid glands that are very sensitive to iodine.* They can develop hypothyroidism as a side effect if they are given iodine in a medication or in a dye such as those used to x-ray the kidneys, gall bladder, or spinal canal. Health food users can similarly, and unknowingly, take in excessive amounts of iodine by eating kelp (seaweed). Hypothyroidism can also develop in patients who receive large amounts of x-rays to the neck area as part of cancer treatment.

DIAGNOSING HYPOTHYROIDISM

If your physician suspects hypothyroidism, he or she will first perform a medical examination to look for the evidence that your thyroid level is low (see above). Next, a blood sample will be obtained. Usually, your blood level of the thyroid hormone *thyroxine* (T_4) will be low. The most important test in making a certain diagnosis of this condition, however, is your TSH blood level, for when your thyroid gland fails, your pituitary begins to produce increased amounts of TSH, as if to stimulate your thyroid more and return it to a normal function. Since your thyroid cannot increase its activity, your blood level of TSH rises and remains high. The

---

*See Chapter 14 for a more complete discussion of lithium and iodine.

demonstration of an increased level of TSH in your blood also provides evidence that your hypothyroidism is due to disease within your thyroid gland and is not a result of inadequate stimulation of your thyroid by a diseased pituitary gland.

If your hypothyroidism is mild and your TSH level is not clearly elevated above normal, your physician may decide to do a *TRH test*. TRH refers to *TSH releasing hormone* and is a brain hormone from the hypothalamus, which normally helps control the release of TSH from your pituitary gland (Figure 17). A normal individual responds to an injection of synthetic TRH by a modest increase in the level of TSH. In contrast, if your thyroid is even slightly underactive, you should show a greater-than-normal increase in serum TSH concentration after TRH is given (Figure 18).

A word might be said about a dangerous recent trend in the lay press to minimize the importance of thyroid

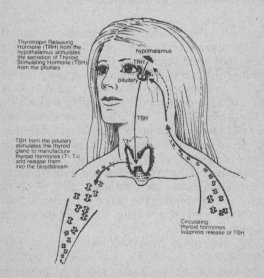

Thyrotropin Releasing Hormone (TRH) from the hypothalamus stimulates the secretion of Thyroid Stimulating Hormone (TSH) from the pituitary

hypothalamus

TRH

pituitary

TSH

TSH from the pituitary stimulates the thyroid gland to manufacture thyroid hormones (T₃ T₄) and release them into the bloodstream

Circulating thyroid hormones suppress release of TSH

Figure 17 The Hypothalamic- Pituitary-Thyroid Axis.

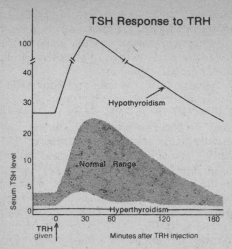

Figure 18 A hypothyroid patient responds to an injection of TRH by producing excessive amounts of TSH.

blood tests in the diagnosis and management of hypothyroidism. The thyroid tests available 20 or 30 years ago were simply not specific enough to tell if a person was truly hypothyroid. Very accurate and relatively inexpensive tests *are* available today, however, and they should *always* be used by your physician to help make a diagnosis of hypothyroidism. Such a diagnosis should *never* be based solely on complaints of weight gain, fatigue, or infertility, or on such nonspecific findings as dry skin or a low body temperature. Well-informed physicians do not start patients on thyroid medication until blood tests confirming the diagnosis are obtained. Such blood tests are essential in determining the cause and severity of the hypothyroidism, and in assessing the adequacy of thyroid therapy.

Finally, since most hypothyroidism is caused by chronic lymphocytic thyroiditis, a sample of your blood can be checked for the *antibodies* that may appear as a clue to the presence of this type of thyroid inflammation.

THE TREATMENT OF HYPOTHYROIDISM

Hypothyroidism is treated with thyroid hormone tablets. Fortunately, thyroid hormones are normal body substances, and therefore, you will not be allergic to them. Moreover, since the hormones are not destroyed by stomach juices, they can be given by mouth. Finally, if taken correctly, thyroid hormones have no unwanted effects on any body tissues.

Today, many different thyroid hormone preparations are manufactured. For many years, however, the only thyroid hormone medications available were made from animal thyroid glands.* These preparations were very useful, but unfortunately they contain not only thyroxine (T_4), but also a second more rapidly acting thyroid hormone, triiodothyronine (T_3).

We prefer to administer thyroid hormone tablets that do not contain T_3 for two reasons. First, the body normally makes T_3 from T_4; in fact, much of our T_4 is changed into T_3 under normal circumstances, as it is used by the body. Second, the blood T_3 level can become abnormally high after taking medication that contains T_3. The abnormally high T_3 level can cause a rapid pulse and increase the workload of the heart, which can be dangerous for anyone with underlying heart disease. For these reasons, therefore, most physicians now treat hypothyroidism with tablets of pure T_4 rather than tablets that contain both T_4 and T_3.

A comment about T_4 tablets must be made. There is an increasing tendency today to use generic forms of drugs as opposed to more expensive forms sold under a trade name. Although generic drugs are generally less expensive, generic thyroid preparations have always presented a problem of unreliable potency. Recently,

*These medications are still available and are sold as Proloid or desiccated thyroid.

tests conducted in the United States have shown this same variability of potency in generic T_4 tablets.[11] In fact, only two kinds of T_4 tablets were found to be consistently reliable: *Levothroid* and *Synthroid*.* Therefore, the authors prescribe only these two thyroid preparations at this time. These tablets have a nearly identical "color code" (thyroxine tablets of different potencies come in different colors), which helps to avoid confusion about thyroid hormone dosage (see Table 1).

TABLE 1

Comparative Availability of Thyroxine Preparations in the United States and Canada

Thyroxine Dosage	Tablet Color	Synthroid	Available as Levothroid	Eltroxin
25 micrograms	orange	yes	yes	no
50	white	yes	yes	yes
75	lavender	yes	no	no
100	yellow	yes	yes	yes
125	Synthroid-tan	yes	yes	no
125	Levothroid-purple	yes	yes	no
150	blue	yes	yes	yes
175	turquoise	no	yes	no
200	pink	yes	yes	yes
300	green	yes	yes	yes

Synthroid is available in the United States and Canada, while Levothroid is marketed only in the United States and Eltroxin only in Canada.

When thyroxine tablets first began to be used, physicians thought that 100 micrograms of T_4 was equivalent in potency to a one-grain tablet of desiccated thyroid or Proloid. In practice, however, we have found that these older preparations are not reliably potent. Therefore, when changing a patient from a desiccated thyroid tablet to T_4, we usually start at a slightly lower dose of T_4. For example, someone who has taken two or three grains of thyroid may be started on 100 to 150 micrograms of thy-

*In Canada, Synthroid and Eltroxin are reliable preparations of thyroxine (T_4).

roxine. In fact, few patients *ever* need more than 100 to 200 micrograms of thyroxine per day.

Even when hypothyroidism is severe, a few months of thyroid treatment should lead to complete recovery and a return to good health. At that time, your physician will probably measure your blood levels of T_4 and TSH to be sure that your dosage of thyroid hormone is correct. If you are taking too much T_4 your blood level of T_4 may be above the normal range. On the other hand, if your dose of T_4 is too low, your blood level of T_4 will be low and your TSH still will be above the normal range.

The smooth control of thyroid hormone level that physicians achieve by using pure thyroxine preparations is due to the slow rate at which thyroxine is used up by the body. In fact, if a normal person's thyroid suddenly stopped working, it would take about seven days for the body to use up just half of the T_4 already in the blood. Therefore, if you are hypothyroid and taking thyroxine tablets to correct your thyroid deficiency, you will not feel suddenly sick even if you stop your thyroxine tablets abruptly. Furthermore, because you won't notice a sudden change in the way you feel, you may incorrectly assume that your thyroid condition no longer exists and you may stop taking your medication entirely. Unfortunately, when your hypothyroidism does recur, its onset may be so gradual that you may not realize that you are becoming ill again until your symptoms are pronounced.

In hypothyroidism due to chronic lymphocytic thyroiditis, there is also a need for good "family follow-up" since this illness, like hyperthyroidism due to Graves' disease, is a genetically transmitted disease. The genes for it came from either your mother or your father (or rarely from both). Therefore, older members on the side of the family affected should be checked for thyroid problems as well as for certain associated medical conditions. These relationships are discussed in Chapter 8.

If you are hypothyroid, it is important that you see your physician periodically for checkups. Since most hypothyroidism tends to get worse progressively over months and years, a dose of thyroid hormone that was correct several years ago may well be inadequate as thyroid replacement now. Therefore, your physician will probably want to measure your serum T_4 and TSH periodically to be sure that a change in hormone dosage is not indicated.

A word might be said about treating certain of the less common causes of thyroid failure. For example, subacute thyroiditis, which may be due to a viral infection, may only temporarily decrease thyroid function. If a patient needs any thyroxine treatment for a transient hypothyroid condition, it should be only a matter of weeks or months before he or she can stop the drug and remain well. And when hypothyroidism is due to iodine ingestion or an antithyroid drug, simply stopping or decreasing the dose of the drug may be all that is required. In every such instance, your physician has the necessary tests available as a guide in properly taking care of you.

As we have already suggested, many patients who were started on thyroid medication years ago may not have needed thyroid treatment then, and may not need it now. Thyroid testing available today makes it possible for us to find out safely and easily whether such patients can stop their thyroid tablets and remain well.

If you took thyroid hormone treatment for many years and want to know if you still need the medication, please ask your physician for guidance rather than stopping treatment on your own. If you both agree to a trial without thyroid tablets, your physician will probably just measure your blood level of TSH six weeks after you have stopped the medication. If your TSH level is normal, you do not need thyroxine treatment, for your own thyroid function is fine.

SOME OTHER KINDS OF HYPOTHYROIDISM

Since the pituitary gland at the base of your brain controls and stimulates your thyroid, a tumor or other problem that involves the pituitary can cause "secondary" thyroid failure. Since your pituitary also controls other glands, including your reproductive organs and adrenal glands, it is usually an easy matter for your physician to tell if this is the case. For example, a woman with *secondary (pituitary) hypothyroidism* will usually stop menstruating when her diseased pituitary gland stops stimulating her ovaries properly. Physicians have at their disposal both x-ray techniques and laboratory tests to evaluate the function of your pituitary gland as well as your thyroid. If there is indeed a pituitary problem, you will probably require treatment for other hormonal deficiencies in addition to the thyroid. If your pituitary fails because of a tumor, specific treatment may be directed at the pituitary gland itself. Fortunately, pituitary tumors respond to both surgical and radiation treatment.* Just as with primary hypothyroidism, you will need careful and prolonged follow-up, for in addition to thyroid hormone requirements, the amounts of other hormones you take may vary with time. Thus, periodic blood tests and x-rays of the pituitary area will probably be recommended by your physician.

The pituitary is itself under the control of the hypothalamus, an even higher center within the brain. In very rare instances, disease in the region of the hypothalamus has caused the pituitary to fail and, in turn, has caused thyroid and other glandular problems. Although this condition of *tertiary hypothyroidism* looks very much

---

*It should also be mentioned that hypothyroidism may appear *after* treatment of a pituitary tumor, if the treatment damages the pituitary in such a way that it can no longer make enough TSH to stimulate the thyroid properly.

like secondary hypothyroidism, physicians can distinguish one form from another by means of careful testing. Treatment is similar to that given when the problem is in the pituitary gland, and it must include correction not only of the hypothyroidism, but also of the other glandular deficiencies as well.

In summary, hypothyroidism is almost always due to disease within your thyroid gland that causes a decrease in the production of thyroid hormone. Good tests are available to diagnose the condition accurately, and treatment with thyroxine should restore you to good health. Because the condition runs in families, some of your relatives should be checked for thyroid problems by their own physicians (see chapter 8).

CHAPTER SEVEN

Inflammation of the Thyroid

Hashimoto's Disease and Other Forms of Thyroiditis

"Thyroiditis" is the general term used to describe three different disorders in which the thyroid gland becomes inflamed. Most commonly, the inflammation takes the form of a chronic, progressive disease known as chronic lymphocytic thyroiditis or *Hashimoto's disease*. This condition may be so mild that it may go unnoticed for many years, but eventually it may destroy so much thyroid tissue that hypothyroidism develops. In a second type of thyroiditis, the thyroid becomes temporarily inflamed, usually in association with a viral infection. This condition is known as *subacute thyroiditis* or *DeQuervain's disease*.* Finally, and *very* rarely, the thyroid may become suddenly and dramatically inflamed with a bacterial infection. This condition is referred to as *acute suppurative† thyroiditis*. Since these three forms of thyroiditis are completely different disorders—each with a different cause, clinical course, and treatment—they will be considered separately.

*Hashimoto and DeQuervain are the names of physicians who have been so honored because of their important contribution to our understanding of these forms of thyroiditis.

†The term *suppurative* refers to the presence of a bacterial infection.

75

Chronic Lymphocytic Thyroiditis (Hashimoto's Disease)

Hashimoto's disease appears to be an inherited condition. As with Graves' disease, you probably must inherit a gene or set of genes to be *able* to develop this disorder. However, even though you may inherit this genetic tendency, you still may never actually develop the disease itself. Therefore, there must be other factors involved to produce this condition.

Like those of Graves' disease, these other causative factors include your sex hormones, your age, and your body's immune system. Thus, women are affected at least nine times more often than men, and although you may develop this form of thyroiditis in childhood or adolescence, it is most commonly diagnosed after the age of forty, for this is when affected patients usually become hypothyroid. Your body's immune system seems to play a role in the production of the thyroid inflammation and tissue destruction that occurs in chronic lymphocytic thyroiditis. Substances known as *autoantibodies*, made by certain white blood cells called *lymphocytes*, appear in your blood in this condition. Although we do not yet fully understand how these antibodies work, it seems likely that some of them have the capacity to damage thyroid tissue. When enough tissue has been destroyed, your thyroid hormone production falls below normal, and symptoms of hypothyroidism appear.

This form of thyroiditis is common, and its incidence may well be increasing. A population survey in Minnesota carried out by physicians at Mayo Clinic between 1935 and 1944 reported that, among women, new cases of chronic lymphocytic thyroiditis occurred at a rate of 6.5 per 100,000 women per year. When the same Minnesota population group was studied again in 1965–67, this "annual incidence" of the disorder had increased to 69 per 100,000 women per year. Autopsy studies show evidence of thyroiditis in up to 6 percent of individuals who supposedly had no symptoms or signs of a thyroid problem during life. Indeed, this figure is more in accord with modern estimates of the prevalence of this disease.

One way that physicians have tried to estimate the prevalence of Hashimoto's disease is by testing groups of people for hypothyroidism. As noted above, this form of thyroiditis damages thyroid tissue and leads to thyroid failure. The most sensitive test for hypothyroidism is a blood test that measures the level of the pituitary's thyroid stimulating hormone (TSH). When TSH tests are carried out on large numbers of people, we find that about 10 percent of women and 4 percent of men over the age of fifty have an elevated blood level of TSH, suggesting that the true prevalence of chronic thyroiditis among women may be higher than previously suspected, while its prevalence in men is somewhat lower. Put another way, *at least* one woman in ten will probably develop Hashimoto's disease in her lifetime. Each of these women has the potential of developing subsequent hypothyroidism and should be watched for the development of that complication. Fortunately, only a small percentage may actually need any form of treatment.

If you develop this condition, your thyroid inflammation will probably be so mild that at first you won't even know that anything is wrong. The first indication of a problem may be a goiter: You will notice a gradual painless enlargement of your thyroid gland. During this period, your thyroid gland is becoming infiltrated with lymphocytes, which start gradual thyroid destruction and scarring that result in subsequent thyroid failure. If the function of your thyroid decreases to the point that your gland can no longer make a normal amount of thyroid hormone, symptoms of hypothyroidism appear, and you may begin to look and feel sick for the first time. At this point, the destruction of your thyroid may be so extensive that very little normal thyroid tissue remains.

When hypothyroidism occurs, you probably will feel sluggish and "rundown," but the disease progresses slowly, so you may not realize that anything is wrong. Constipation, leg cramps, hair loss and mental dullness may appear, together with other symptoms and signs of thyroid failure already outlined in Chapter 6. However, since chronic lymphocytic thyroiditis tends to be a progressive condition, your thyroid hormone level will probably continue to fall, causing your symptoms of hypothyroidism to worsen until, it is hoped, your disease is recognized and treated.

If you visit your doctor and are found to have hypothyroidism and a goiter, with no history of a past problem with your thyroid, your physician will probably suspect that you have chronic lymphocytic thyroiditis. This diagnosis becomes even more likely if other members of your family have had overactive or underactive thyroids. Your physician can confirm the presence of hypothyroidism by means of a blood test that shows a low level of thyroid hormone (T_4) and a high blood level of thyroid stimulating hormone. The elevated TSH level is the more important test, for it is more sensitive and proves that your thyroid, not your pituitary, has failed (see chapter 6). A radioiodine uptake and scan of your thyroid are so variable that they are not usually of much help in trying to diagnose this condition, though the scan may demonstrate the generalized nature of the thyroiditis by showing a patchy uptake of radioiodine throughout your thyroid gland (Figure 19). On the other hand, the demonstration of antithyroid antibodies in your blood provides strong evidence that thyroiditis is present. Absolute proof of the diagnosis can be obtained only by biopsy of your thyroid gland and microscopic examination of the tissue obtained. Fortunately, a biopsy is rarely necessary.

In the early stages of this condition, while your thyroid hormone levels remain normal, you should feel well and no treatment is required. If your thyroid is large, however, your physician may prescribe thyroid hormone tablets in an effort to reduce the size of your goiter (see Chapter 3 for a discussion of suppression therapy).

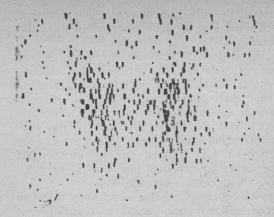

Figure 19   An artist's rendition of a scan shows chronic lymphocytic thyroiditis usually produces a patchy pattern of radioiodine throughout the thyroid.

Later, when your thyroid hormone level falls below normal and symptoms of hypothyroidism appear, thyroid hormone treatment is clearly indicated. As explained in detail in Chapter 6, your physician will probably prescribe thyroxine (T_4) tablets once a day in gradually increasing dosages until your blood level of TSH falls to normal. Since this condition is progressive, lifelong follow-up is essential, but it usually amounts to no more than your physician's examining your thyroid and testing your blood levels of T_4 and TSH at the time of your periodic health checkup.

SUBACUTE THYROIDITIS (DEQUERVAIN'S DISEASE)

Subacute thyroiditis often follows a viral infection. Many different viruses are associated with this condition, including those that cause mumps and measles, as well as some of those that cause the common cold. Since few people who develop a viral infection ever have evidence of thyroid inflammation, subacute thyroiditis is a relatively rare condition.

Typically, symptoms of subacute thyroiditis begins about two weeks after the first signs of viral illness. When they start, you will probably look and feel as though you had an infection, with a painful enlarged thyroid, fever, muscle aches, and fatigue. An astute patient may notice that it is the *thyroid* that hurts in subacute thyroiditis, rather than the *inside* of the throat as is the case with most sore throats. Because the thyroid pain seems to spread toward your jaw or ears, you may think you have a bad tooth or ear infection.

The history of a recent viral illness, followed by fever and an enlarged tender thyroid should make your physician suspect subacute thyroiditis. A high red blood cell sedimentation rate, indicating the presence of an inflammatory condition, is important evidence that the diagnosis is correct. In the test for sedimentation rate, we measure how fast red blood cells settle in a narrow test tube. If you have an inflammatory condition such as this form of thyroiditis, the red blood cells usually settle faster than normal.

Your blood level of thyroid hormone is often elevated in the first weeks of the illness as thyroid hormones escape from your inflamed gland. Unlike hyperthyroidism caused by Graves' disease, your radioactive iodine uptake is very low in this phase of subacute thyroiditis. Thus, these two forms of hyperthyroidism can be differentiated from each other. Later, when your gland becomes depleted of hormones, low blood levels of thyroid hormones may be found with an associated elevation of your blood TSH level. Ultimately, you can expect to recover completely and stay well.

Fortunately, this disorder is self-limited and usually responds readily to medical treatment. Since you may have two different problems, two types of treatment may be required. Your fever and thyroid pain are usually controlled by aspirin alone. In rare instances, however, these symptoms are so severe that the inflammation must be treated with a steroid medication such as cortisone or prednisone. The two lobes of the thyroid may be involved together or at different times, but in either instance the condition rarely lasts longer than four to six weeks.

The changing level of thyroid hormone in your blood may also require treatment. During the early hyperthyroid phase of the disease, a *beta adrenergic blocking drug* like atenolol or propranolol is sometimes prescribed to decrease the effect of too much thyroid hormone on your body. Weeks later, if the thyroid hormone level falls below normal, supplementary thyroxine (T_4) tablets may be prescribed until your own thyroid begins working again. Ultimately, you can expect total and complete recovery within five to six months.

Spontaneously   resolving   hyperthyroidism (see Chapter 5) is a condition that shares several features with subacute thyroiditis and therefore should be mentioned here. Patients with either disorder tend to experience the same progression from *hyper*thyroidism to *hypo*thyroidism and then to normal thyroid function. Unlike patients with subacute thyroiditis, however, patients with SRH lack the signs of thyroid inflammation (pain and fever) and usually have a normal sedimentation rate.

The treatment for spontaneously resolving hyperthyroidism is a beta adrenergic blocking drug like atenolol or propranolol until the hyperthyroid phase of the disease is over. Unfortunately, the disease may recur in some patients, and occasionally it becomes necessary to remove the thyroid surgically in order to cure the condition.

ACUTE SUPPURATIVE THYROIDITIS

This is most often a disease of children but may occur at any age. If you develop this uncommon condition, you will be *very* sick. A bacterial infection is the usual cause of acute suppurative thyroiditis, so you will probably have chills, a very high fever, and hot, tender thyroid; often there is an abscess within the gland.

As with other bacterial infections, antibiotics are required for treatment and local surgical drainage or removal of abscessed tissue may be needed. In spite of the severity of acute suppurative thyroiditis, complete recovery is the usual outcome in this disease.

In summary, although the three forms of thyroiditis all involve inflammation of the thyroid gland, they are quite different disorders. Nevertheless, they all can be readily and easily diagnosed, and they all improve rapidly with the very effective treatments that are available.

SUBACUTE THYROIDITIS

by M. F.

I have been in general good health all my life. I work doing market research and have always had normal energy. As far as I know, neither I nor any other member of my family has ever had a thyroid problem.

I remember that in October 1974 I was feeling well until I got what seemed to be a cold. My throat felt sore and scratchy but the difference this time was a swelling which appeared in the left side of my neck. I became extremely weak, even in the morning when I first got up. There were days when I seemed to have the strength to do some work and light housekeeping, but there were other days when I wanted just to stay in bed. I remember most the throbbing at the bottom of my neck on the left side with pain aching in my left ear at the same time. I felt so sick I saw my doctor, who felt that I might have a strep throat and started treatment with penicillin and aspirin. I felt better within a day, and so well that in four days I stopped the aspirin and continued the penicillin. Much to my surprise I got sick again within a day with a recurrence of my sore throat, swollen neck, and extreme weakness. By this time I was also beginning to notice that my heart was racing. Sometimes it seemed to skip very fast for several minutes, and then suddenly it would stop racing and beat normally again.

I called my doctor, who increased the penicillin. Aspirin was added again, and I soon felt better. Once again, however, when I stopped the aspirin after I felt better my symptoms all returned.

I saw a thyroid specialist on November 20, 1974, who diagnosed my condition as "subacute thyroiditis." He explained that the aspirin was the main drug that was helping me and that there was no sign of any other infection at that time. Aspirin was restarted and within a day my sore throat began to feel better, my strength began to return, and I felt generally improved. I stopped taking the penicillin.

Unfortunately the fast pulse continued, and when the doctor called me to say that my thyroid blood level was high, he said that was causing my heart to race. I was glad that he understood the problem. I took a drug called propranolol four times a day, which slowed the heart rate but which, I understand, did not change the thyroid at all. For about a month and a half I took both aspirin and propranolol and felt fairly well, though not completely cured. During this time, interestingly, the soreness and swelling in my neck moved to the right side, while the left side of my neck became more normal. After about two months, my thyroid level dropped and I began to feel sluggish and cold and had some leg cramps, too. My doctor prescribed thyroid hormone tablets at that time, which raised my thyroid level to normal and returned me to good health. I stopped the thyroid pills after a month because by that time my thyroid had completely healed itself, and after that I felt normal without any medicine at all.

If I could give advice to other patients with this condition, I would say that aspirin seems to help a lot in this condition. If your doctor says you need propranolol, take it regularly too, since each pill only works for a short time. Third, since the thyroid hormone levels changed in my condition, they may change in yours. Check with your doctor as often as the doctor feels necessary until you are well. Fourth, be relieved that you have a condition that should go away completely and leave you with a normal thyroid gland and good health.

CHAPTER EIGHT

If You Have Graves' Disease or Hashimoto's Thyroiditis, What About Your Family?

Graves' disease is an inherited condition, and your tendency to have it was given to you in genes from your mother or father. That parent, and some other relatives on that side of your family, already may have had an overactive thyroid like yours. On the other hand, they may not be aware of any thyroid problem in the past or at present. But those relatives who share your genetic tendency toward Graves' disease may have an unrecognized thyroid abnormality that you can help discover.

If your younger relatives with the inherited tendency to Graves' disease have a thyroid problem, it is likely to be an overactive gland like yours (Figure 43). Usually they are not hard to recognize, for their complaints will be fairly obvious, and will include symptoms you have had yourself, such as nervousness, palpitations, shaky hands, weight loss, and perhaps prominent eyes as well. On the other hand, other relatives—especially those over the age of fifty, like your parents and grandparents —may have hypothyroidism (Figure 44). Since symptoms of hypothyroidism may be mild (feeling cold, tired, a lack of energy, etc.), these older relatives may just accept those symptoms as signs of "getting old." Instead, if their symptoms are due to thyroid failure, they would feel better and be healthier if they were given treatment with thyroid hormone. Their thyroids may be failing for two reasons. First, they may have had unrecognized hyperthyroidism in earlier years and may now be progressing to hypothyroidism in the natural course of their disease. On the other hand, their thyroid glands may be failing because of Hashimoto's disease—chronic lymphocytic thyroiditis. This condition, which tends to occur in families in which other relatives have Graves' disease,[12] produces gradual scarring within the thyroid gland and may lead to hypothyroidism if enough thyroid tissue is destroyed by the process.

There is another side of this too. You and all your relatives with this inherited tendency to thyroid trouble also have a greater than normal chance of developing certain other conditions. These involve many different parts of your body, and include the following:

HAIR—Prematurely gray—anyone who finds a gray hair before the age of 30 years is considered "prematurely gray."

—Patchy hair loss (*alcopecia areata*)—often mild and temporary, but may be extensive and long-lasting. It usually appears in the scalp but may involve other hairy areas, such as the beard.

SKIN—White patches on the skin (*vitiligo*)—white areas that are painless and often placed symmetrically in places like the knuckles, wrists, elbows, and neck.

BLOOD—Anemia (a decrease in red blood cells) due to a lack of Vitamin B_{12} (*pernicious anemia*) and *not* any of the anemias due to other causes.

JOINTS—*Rheumatoid arthritis*—usually a symmetrical, deforming arthritis involving especially the hands, wrists, and feet. Morning stiffness is a common complaint.

EYES—Protrusion of the eyes (*exophthalmos*). If the condition is mild, elevation of the eyelids may be all that is noted (Figure 50).

METABOLISM—*Diabetes mellitus* ("sugar diabetes"), which usually starts at a young age and requires insulin treatment.

We are not trying to imply that everyone who has diabetes or turns prematurely gray will have a thyroid problem. Rather we are saying that these disorders tend to occur in patients with Graves' disease and Hashimoto's disease, and in their relatives, with greater frequency than in the general population. The implications of this observation are twofold: First, physicians will tend to watch you and your family more carefully for the development of one of these problems that may require treatment. Pernicious anemia is such a condition, and it can be controlled simply by a monthly injection of Vitamin B_{12} (see Chapter 9). Second, some of these conditions are more obvious than hypothyroidism and their presence can help you and your physician know which of your older relatives should be tested for that thyroid problem. Not everyone in your family should be tested, for that would be a waste of time and money for a lot of your relatives. But we can, and probably should, encourage those that are at greatest risk for a thyroid problem to see their family physician.

A search for thyroid and related conditions among the family of a 24-year-old woman who has Graves' disease is shown in the hypothetical family tree in this chapter (see Figure 20).

The inheritance of thyroid disease in this family appears to have come from the mother's father down through the mother to the patient. Therefore, the patient's maternal aunts and uncles should be evaluated for a thyroid condition since they all have received half their genes from their hypothyroid father. The uncle with vitiligo and a goiter and the aunt with diabetes are perhaps more likely to develop hypothyroidism in later years than is the patient's apparently healthy aunt, who has no signs of thyroid disease or a related condition. The patient's mother is "at risk" for a thyroid problem not only because of her prematurely gray hair but also because she has a hyperthyroid daughter.

Some of the hyperthyroid patient's brothers and sisters and one of her children are already showing signs that they have inherited a tendency toward thyroid disease, but only one sister has actually developed a problem (hyperthyroidism) requiring treatment.

WHO SHOULD BE TESTED?

Since *hypo*thyroidism tends to be a disease that comes on in later years, we tend to look for that condition only in those relatives who are over the age of fifty and who are on the side of the family that the thyroid tendency came from. In the example that would be the maternal side. We would test them whether they looked and felt sick or not, since hypothyroidism is hard to recognize in many patients, especially if the condition is mild. If younger relatives looked or felt hypothyroid, they could be tested by their physicians too, but we would not recommend this study if they felt well.

Similarly, not everyone need be tested for *hyper*thyroidism on the mother's side in our hypothetical family. When that condition occurs, it is usually fairly obvious,

DIRECTIONS:

O = FEMALE   □ = MALE

THE DIAGRAM BELOW REPRESENTS YOUR
FAMILY TREE, AND WILL HELP YOU FIND
OUT WHO IN YOUR FAMILY IS "AT RISK"
FOR A THYROID DISORDER.

1. WRITE THE AGE OF EACH LIVING
    RELATIVE IN THE O OR □ BELOW.

2. FOR RELATIVES WHO HAVE DIED, WRITE
    THEIR AGE AT DEATH IN THE O OR □
    AND ADD A (†) AFTER THE NUMBER.

3. FOR RELATIVES WHO HAVE HAD ONE
    OR MORE OF THESE DISEASES, WRITE
    THE APPROPRIATE SYMBOL UNDER
    THE O OR □.

EXAMPLE:

A WOMAN WHO DIED AT AGE 65
AND HAD VITILIGO AND DIABETES,
AND BEGAN TO NOTICE GRAY
HAIR BEFORE AGE 30 WOULD BE
SHOWN AS FOLLOWS:

vitiligo
diabetes
premature gray hair

THYROID AND ASSOCIATED CONDITIONS

THYROID:
    overactive
    underactive
    thyroiditis
    goiter (enlarged thyroid)

HAIR:
    prematurely gray (any gray before age 30)
    alopecia areata (patchy hair loss)

SKIN:
    vitiligo (white skin spots)

BLOOD:
    pernicious anemia (anemia due to lack of Vitamin B_{12}
    and NOT other kinds of anemia)

JOINTS:
    rheumatoid arthritis (and NOT other forms
    of arthritis)

EYES:
    exophthalmos (protruding eyes)

METABOLISM:
    diabetes mellitus ("sugar diabetes") which requires
    insulin treatment

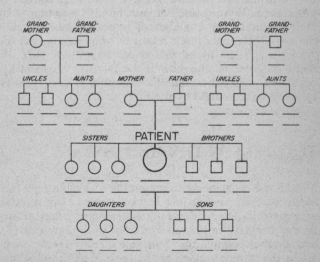

Figure 20 A scheme to help you trace your own family
tree for thyroid and related conditions.

and we could limit testing to younger or older relatives who had hyperactivity, rapid pulse, or other evidence suggestive of excessive thyroid function.

With that perspective in mind, if you or any of your relatives have a thyroid or related problem you can examine your family to see if you can tell who should be checked for *hypo*thyroidism or *hyper*thyroidism. In carrying out the evaluation of your family, you probably will find that several relatives on one side of the family will have had either a thyroid disorder or a thyroid-associated condition. In contrast, those relatives on the other side of the family probably will have had few, if any, of the disorders. Figure 21 is a scheme that we have worked out that can help you trace various thyroid and related conditions through your family tree.

We would recommend that everyone over the age of fifty on the "thyroid side" of your family be examined by their physician for evidence of hypothyroidism. Below the age of fifty, only those relatives who feel sluggish and "rundown" need to be tested for hypothyroidism. Finally, relatives on the side of the family who seem hyperactive (fast pulse, increased sweating, nervousness, etc.) can be examined by their physicians for evidence of hyperthyroidism.

TESTING FOR THYROID DISEASE

In addition to a medical examination, simple tests are available that can tell whether someone is hypothyroid or hyperthyroid. A single blood sample, taken at any time of the day, can be analyzed for both thyroxine (T_4) and thyroid stimulating hormone (TSH) levels. Normally, the pituitary gland at the base of the brain stimulates the thyroid gland with small quantities of TSH, causing the thyroid to produce T_4. However, if thyroid failure occurs, the pituitary senses less T_4 in the blood and makes more TSH. Thus, the combination of a low T_4 and a high TSH in the blood is an important sensitive indication of the presence of hypothyroidism. If hyperthyroidism is present, a blood test will usually show an elevated thyroid hormone level. If the level is in a borderline range, more sensitive tests can be done that will tell if the condition is present (see Chapter 4).

HOW SERIOUS ARE THESE CONDITIONS?

As we focus attention on the inheritance of thyroid disease within a family, we risk alarming patients needlessly about possible illnesses in their parents and children. Actually, thyroid troubles rarely cause serious or life-threatening problems. A person who is hypothyroid can have mild hypothyroidism for years with no symptoms except, perhaps, mild fatigue. Similarly, someone who is hyperthyroid can look and feel perfectly well (though perhaps somewhat hyperenergetic).

We are calling attention to these patterns of inheritance in an effort to find patients with mild conditions and thus improve their quality of life. For example, an older person with hypothyroidism may well have more energy and productivity if his or her low thyroid levels are increased. And a young person with mild hyperthyroidism will usually feel calmer and be physically stronger if that condition is controlled.

In another way, a search for disease might help an older relative on the "thyroid side" of your family, if he or she were discovered to have pernicious anemia. This condition, like hypothyroidism, can come on so slowly that it can remain unrecognized, yet cause sluggishness due to the anemia (low blood count) or clumsiness and loss of balance due to involvement of the nervous system. It is the authors' custom to test for pernicious anemia by means of a blood test for Vitamin B_{12} in patients over the age of sixty who have had Graves' disease or Hashimoto's disease, or who are on the "thyroid side" of such a family. A full discussion of pernicious anemia (as well as the other conditions that are associated with Graves' disease and Hashimoto's disease) can be found in Chapter 9.

WHAT WILL THE TREATMENT BE?

When found, an underactive thyroid is usually treated by the patient's physician with small amounts of thyroid hormone supplementation given as a thyroxine tablet* to be taken once a day. Starting doses in those individuals over fifty years of age must be small, since some older persons do not tolerate sudden big changes in their thyroid hormone levels. Thereafter, the dose is increased every month or so until the T_4 and TSH are normal.

Since the symptoms of hyperthyroidism are due to the presence of too much thyroid hormone in the body, treatment of that condition is aimed at reducing the production of hormone by the thyroid gland. This can be done by medicines that affect the thyroid. Alternatively, it is possible to decrease the production of thyroid hormone either by removing part of the gland in an operation or by destroying some of the thyroid tissue with radioactive iodine. In practice, treatment is individualized by physicians, and depends upon each patient's particular circumstances, including age and other health problems.

---

*According to medical tests on thyroid hormone tablets, the most reliably potent forms of thyroxine sold in the United States are Levothroid and Synthroid. In Canada, both Synthroid and Eltroxin are reliable preparations. We do NOT recommend *generic* prescriptions for thyroid hormone because the thyroxine content of such tablets may vary.

WHAT HAVE YOU LEARNED?

We have prepared this guide as a part of an ongoing effort to reach people who need treatment for thyroid disease and to educate them about their disorder.

We hope that you decide to carry out this thyroid search within your family, and that you will let your family physician know the results. Your physician should be able to aide you if you have questions about how to do the search or about which relatives should be tested for thyroid problems.

CHAPTER NINE

Graves' Disease, Hashimoto's Thyroiditis, and Some Related Conditions

Addison's Disease, Allergy, Pernicious Anemia, Rheumatoid Arthritis, Diabetes, and Disorders of the Eyes, Hair, Liver, Muscles, and Skin

> For a long period I had from time to time met with a very remarkable form of general anaemia, occurring without any discoverable cause whatever ... The leading and characteristic features of the morbid state to which I would direct attention are, anaemia, general languor and debility, remarkable feebleness of the heart's action, irritability of the stomach, and a peculiar change of colour in the skin, occurring in connection with a diseased condition of the "suprarenal capsules."
>
> —Thomas Addison (1855)

Thomas Addison believed that he was describing the features of a disease caused by failure of two glands located above the kidneys, now known as the *adrenal glands*, which make *cortisone* and other steroid hormones. Actually, his descriptions suggest that, in addition to *adrenal failure*, some of his patients also had *pernicious anemia*, a blood condition caused by a deficiency of Vitamin B_{12}. It is not surprising that some of Addison's patients had both diseases, for we now know

94

that there is a slight tendency for the two conditions to occur together.*

From time to time, physicians have recognized similar relationships, in which diseases occur together more often than chance alone would allow. In 1926, M. B. Schmidt, a physician in Germany, described two patients in whom both the adrenal and thyroid glands had failed.* Since then, more than 125 patients with both disorders have been described, enough to make us realize that something more than an "accident of nature" makes this rare combination happen.

In several places in this book we have commented on the relationship between Graves' disease and Hashimoto's disease, which tend to occur in the same families, sometimes in the same patients, and which may even be different presentations of a single disease process. This chapter is about the other conditions that tend to occur in patients with Graves' disease and Hashimoto's disease, and in their relatives as well. Some, like the prominent eyes of Graves' disease known as *exophthalmos*, have been well-studied and their relationship to thyroid problems carefully examined. Others, such as some of the associated skin disorders, are less well understood in regard to their relationship to the thyroid.

This chapter is not about those bodily changes that occur due to high or low thyroid hormone levels. High hormone levels, for example, can raise your upper eyelids, make your skin soft and smooth, and cause your hair to become fine and delicate. The high hormone levels do not, however, cause your eyes to protrude, make white patches of *vitiligo* appear on your skin, or produce the patchy baldness we call *alopecia areata*. The latter problems are diseases in their own right and are the subject of this chapter.

These are not, in general, serious problems about

---

*In honor of Dr. Addison, adrenal failure is known as Addison's disease and pernicious anemia is sometimes referred to as Addisonian anemia.

which thyroid patients should be concerned. Many, like *alopecia areata*, do not need treatment, for they tend to go away after a period of time. Others, like *pernicious anemia* or *vitiligi*, can be cured or controlled by appropriate treatment. Some, like *Addison's disease*, are so uncommon that even thyroid specialists rarely see a patient with this condition. Nevertheless, we believe there should be a place in this book to which patients with Graves' disease or Hashimoto's disease could refer if they discover that they or one of their relatives has one of these problems.

ADRENAL GLAND FAILURE (ADDISON'S DISEASE)

Your adrenal glands make *cortisone* and other *steroid hormones*, which are released into your blood stream daily and are especially important in your response to stressful situations. Adrenal failure is an uncommon condition, occurring in only one individual per 100,000 of the population. In some patients with Addison's disease, the adrenal glands fail due to damage caused by tuberculosis, and these patients have no special tendency to thyroid failure. Patients who develop Addison's disease in association with Hashimoto's disease are those in whom the adrenal glands fail because of a self-destructive process involving the body's immune system, very much like that which causes thyroid failure in Hashimoto's disease (see Chapter 7).

If your adrenal glands fail, you will experience fatigue, loss of energy, weakness, and darkening of your skin, especially over your joints and inside your mouth. This condition is treated by replacing the hormones that the adrenals no longer make in sufficient amounts (cortisone and related steroid hormones).

ALLERGY

Medical studies done many years ago suggested that some allergic disorders seemed to occur with increased frequency among patients with thyroid problems. Unfortunately, this is an area that has received little study during recent years when thyroid tests have become accurate and specific. Therefore, it is not possible to say whether these conditions are indeed more common in patients with thyroid problems than in the general population. Some patients who have or who have had thyroid problems seem to have a greater than normal tendency to develop hives from time to time. These red itchy welts on the skin do not necessarily come at times when the thyroid is malfunctioning. They generally respond to treatment with antihistamine drugs.

PERNICIOUS ANEMIA

Anemia is a disorder characterized by a decrease in the number of red blood cells that carry oxygen to various body tissues. If you have hypothyroidism, you may also have an associated mild anemia as one manifestation of the general slowing of your body functions that occurs in your condition. The anemia usually causes no symptoms and corrects itself when your hypothyroidism is treated. It is not a separate disease, but is due instead to the low thyroid hormone level.

A more serious type of anemia, known as *pernicious anemia*, is a separate disease that tends to occur in older patients who have or have had Graves' disease or Hashimoto's thyroiditis. This kind of anemia is caused by deficiency of Vitamin B_{12}. Under normal circumstances, cells lining your stomach make a substance known as *intrinsic factor* that enables your body to absorb Vitamin

B_{12} from food. Some individuals lose the ability to absorb Vitamin B_{12}, due to failure of the cells that make intrinsic factor. The damage seems to be caused by a self-destructive process involving the body's immune system, similar to what occurs in Addison's and Hashimoto's diseases. Vitamin B_{12} is an important ingredient in the manufacturing of red blood cells, and if levels of this vitamin fall, anemia may result. Vitamin B_{12} is also important in nourishing your nervous system, so if you develop pernicious anemia, you also may experience numbness and tingling of your hands and feet, loss of balance, and even leg weakness.* It is not clear how many patients who have thyroid functional problems also develop pernicious anemia, though some studies have suggested that as many as 5 percent of patients with Graves' disease and 10 percent of those who have Hashimoto's disease may develop this condition. Since pernicious anemia tends to develop in later years, it is probably even more common in older patients with either condition.

It is the authors' custom to measure the blood level of Vitamin B_{12} in every patient over the age of sixty who has ever had Graves' disease or Hashimoto's thyroiditis. We do this because pernicious anemia is both common and treatable. If your blood level of Vitamin B_{12} appears low or borderline low, another test, known as a *Schilling test*, can be performed. This test demonstrates whether you have difficulty absorbing Vitamin B_{12} from your food. If you do have pernicious anemia, it can be easily treated with Vitamin B_{12} given by intramuscular injection once a month under the supervision of your physician.

---

*Therefore, pernicious anemia is also known as "combined systems disease" because of such associated problems that may occur with the anemia.

ARTHRITIS

Some patients with Graves' or Hashimoto's disease also have a tendency to certain kinds of tendon and joint inflammation. Painful *tendonitis* and *bursitis* of the shoulder, for example, was reported in 6.7 percent of patients but occurs in only about 1.7 percent of the general population.

Rheumatoid arthritis is a more serious disease, in which there is a symmetrical inflammation of many joints of the body, most typically the knuckles, wrists, and elbows. It is also characterized by joint stiffness that is most severe in the morning. Severe rheumatoid arthritis appears to be only slightly more common among patients with thyroid dysfunction than in the general population. If you have hyper- or hypothyroidism you may notice mild morning joint pain and stiffness. If so, like patients with rheumatoid arthritis, you can benefit from treatment with heat, aspirin, and related drugs. On the other hand, some hypothyroid patients have joint pain and stiffness that improves when they are treated with thyroid medication.

DIABETES MELLITUS

Among patients with Graves' or Hashimoto's diseases and their relatives, there is an increased incidence of the type of diabetes that begins in children or young adults and needs to be treated with insulin (so-called *juvenile onset diabetes*). Although it is tempting to assume that both are due to self-destructive influences that damage the thyroid and the pancreas respectively, the two disorders do not necessarily both occur in the same individuals. However, if you do have both conditions at once, an overactive thyroid will often make your diabetes more severe and more difficult to control with insulin.

Treatment of your thyroid problem, in that case, should make your diabetes easier to control.

DYSLEXIA

On the basis of research done largely in the last five years, it appears likely that learning disabilities (dyslexia) are more common in families in which some one has had hyper- or hypothyroidism or Hashimoto's disease than in the general population.

Children with dyslexia may have a variety of problems, including delays in physical or speech development, poor spelling or handwriting, stuttering, right-left confusion, and reversals of numbers or letters. They may be good at math or have the "gift of gab" and are often especially gifted in other ways, including athletics, art, and music. On the other hand, they may have real difficulty reading. Therefore, though these children are usually very bright, poor academic performance is not uncommon and may lead to loss of self-esteem. The condition occurs more commonly in males than females, and affected children are often left-handed or ambidextrous.

Therefore, if you or someone in your family has thyroid dysfunction or chronic thyroiditis and there are children in the family with these sorts of learning problems, you would do well to have them checked by a specialist in learning disabilities, who is obtainable through your school or family physician.

Dyslexia is treatable anytime—the earlier the better —and the academic improvement in special-help programs may be striking. Remember that the learning disabilities are not *caused* by thyroid problems and, in fact, are usually seen in males, while the related thyroid troubles tend to occur in the females in the family.

EYE ENLARGEMENT AND INFLAMMATION

Elevation of the upper eyelids may occur in anyone with hyperthyroidism from any cause, anytime the blood level of thyroid hormone is above normal. For example, someone who is hyperthyroid because of too much thyroid hormone medication may have raised upper eyelids causing his or her eyes to *appear* enlarged or staring. In this situation, however, the eyes do not actually protrude.

If you have Graves' disease you may develop protrusion and inflammation of your eyes without there being any evidence of infection. It is likely to begin about the time your thyroid becomes overactive, but it may precede your hyperthyroidism or occur years after your thyroid function has become normal. Very rarely, the eye disorder may occur without your having any obvious abnormality of thyroid function at *any* time in your life.

More serious eye problems occur only in patients with Graves' disease and (less commonly) Hashimoto's thyroiditis. The severity of these conditions is unrelated to the blood level of thyroid hormone. Instead, if you develop this problem, your eye symptoms and signs will depend on the type and the extent of your inflammatory eye condition. If the condition is mild, you may have only redness and irritation of your eyes. On the other hand, in those rare instances when the inflammation is more severe your eyes may protrude, you may have double vision, and your sight may be threatened.

It should be pointed out that the thyroid eye disease does not necessarily progress in an orderly fashion from mild to severe in any given patient. In fact, a rapid decrease in vision can occur due to pressure upon the optic nerve in a patient with minimal swelling of the eyelids. For this reason, if you have Graves' disease and begin to show signs of eye trouble, you should have a complete eye examination. If your eye involvement is severe, your physician may refer you to an *ophthalmologist* (eye specialist), who will have at his/her disposal all of the equipment needed to evaluate the various eye problems that may occur in Graves' disease. Your vision can be accurately tested. The amount of eye protrusion can be accurately measured with an *exophthalmometer*. The cornea and other tissues of your eye can be examined by the use of a microscopelike instrument known as a *slit lamp*. *Ultrasound* pictures of your eye may be taken, using sound waves in a technique similar to radar. When necessary, special x-rays of your eye socket (*orbit*) can also be obtained.

Treatment of your eye condition will depend upon the kind of eye disease you have and whether it is getting worse. Mild inflammation may be treated simply by elevating the head of your bed at night and by lubricating your eyes with drops of "artificial tears." On the other hand, if you have a severe and rapidly progressive inflammatory condition with double vision or decreased vision, you may require special glasses or treatment with steroids. If your eye tissues continue to swell despite the use of steroid hormones, additional therapy is available. This may include x-ray treatments to the tissues behind the eye or surgery on the bony orbit (*surgical decompression*) to relieve the increased pressure behind your eye.

Fortunately, serious eye problems are rare among thyroid patients. When they do occur, the treatment methods are excellent and are usually successful in improving the problem. Occasionally excessive drooping of the upper or lower eyelids may cause cosmetic problems, but plastic eye surgery can be very helpful for such patients.

HAIR LOSS AND PREMATURELY GRAY HAIR

Changes in thyroid function are associated with a change in the body's use of oxygen (metabolic rate). If the metabolic rate is too high or too low, hair growth may be imperfect. As a result, you may lose some of your hair if your thyroid is either overactive or underactive from any cause. In most cases your hair loss will be generalized and mild, and your hair growth will return to normal as soon as your thyroid problem is controlled.

Patients with Graves' or Hashimoto's disease may notice a *patchy* hair loss instead. This condition, known as *alopecia areata*, is characterized by bald spots anywhere on the body where hair grows, including your scalp and beard. Generally, the condition goes away by itself after several months, regardless of the level of thyroid function and thyroid treatment, but occasionally, such hair loss is permanent.

Physicians have recognized for some time that *prematurely gray hair*, by which we mean hair that *starts* to become gray before age 30, occurs more frequently in patients with thyroid dysfunction than in the general population. This common and easily recognized condition is of course harmless, but is important because it can be helpful to you in tracing the pattern of inheritance of thyroid diseases within your family (Chapter 8).

LIVER DISEASE AND JAUNDICE

Some patients with thyroid dysfunction have an associated tendency to develop *jaundice*, a yellow color of the skin caused by increased blood levels of a substance known as *bilirubin*. Though our knowledge of this relationship is incomplete, some of these patients with

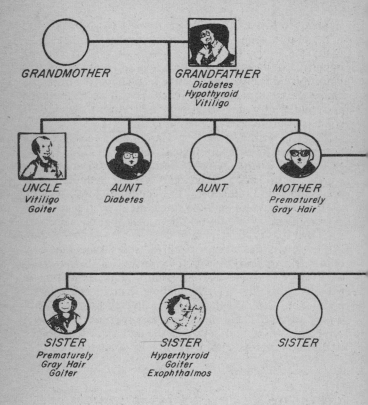

Figure 21 The hypothetical family tree of a 24-year-old woman with hyperthyroidism due to Graves' disease.

Family Search

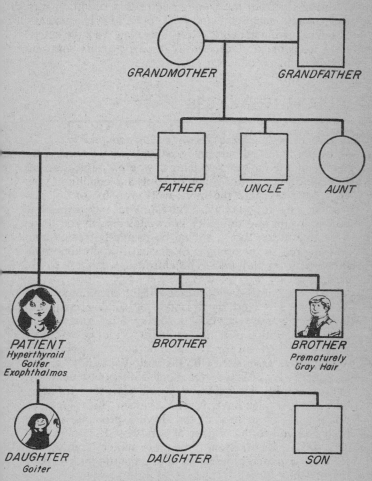

mild jaundice have a harmless condition known as *Gilbert's disease*. In these individuals, jaundice develops from time to time because the liver does not clear bilirubin properly from the blood. Before this condition was understood, such patients were occasionally misdiagnosed as having hepatitis. Now, however, we have better tests available and can easily recognize this form of jaundice when it occurs.

MUSCLE WEAKNESS

A rare muscle disease known as *myasthenia gravis* is about ten times as common in patients with Graves' disease as in the general population, where it affects about 33 people per million. If you develop this condition, you will feel weak, and the more work you try to do, the weaker your muscles will become. You may also have double vision and difficulty in swallowing. If you have hyperthyroidism too, it should be promptly treated and your thyroid level brought to normal, for an abnormal hormone level may cause the muscular weakness to increase.

Periodic paralysis is an exceedingly uncommon condition characterized by episodes of sudden complete temporary paralysis, often occurring after exercise or after consumption of a meal containing a lot of carbohydrate (sugar). A lowering of the blood level of potassium is sometimes associated with the period of paralysis, and in patients so afflicted treatment with potassium may help to control the weakness. Some patients with periodic paralysis also have hyperthyroidism due to Graves' disease. If so, control of the thyroid problem usually brings an end to the attacks of paralysis. For some reason, Asian patients seem to be more subject than others to develop periodic paralysis in association with hyperthyroidism.

SKIN DISORDERS

If your thyroid is overactive from any cause, you will probably notice thinning of your skin and increased sweating. Conversely, if your thyroid is underactive, your skin will probably become thick, rough, and dry. Your skin will return to normal gradually after treatment restores your thyroid hormone level to normal. These problems are due to thyroid dysfunction and are not separate diseases.

Pretibial myxedema is a very rare condition in which reddish, raised, firm, usually nontender lumps develop on the front of the legs and on top of the feet of a few patients with Graves' disease. It arises when substances known as *mucopolysaccharides* are deposited in these areas, but we still do not know why they appear and why only the legs and feet tend to be involved in most patients who have this condition. If you have this problem, it usually responds quite well to treatment with cortisone creams. For greatest effectiveness, these creams can be put on your skin at night under a plastic wrapping material, such as Saran Wrap, held in place by paper adhesive tape.

Vitiligo is a thyroid-related condition in which white patches appear where the skin has lost its normal pigment. It occurs in association with both Graves' disease and Hashimoto's disease and is generally unrelated to the state of the patient's thyroid activity. In most patients, the white spots are small and therefore unnoticed, though in some patients vitiligo may be so extensive as to require dermatologic treatment. In recent years, dermatologists have begun using drugs known as *psoralins*, which, acted upon by sunlight, can increase the amount of skin pigment in most patients with vitiligo. This form of treatment is developing so rapidly that patients with vitiligo who desire information about available treatments should consult a dermatologist.

One of the most common skin-related symptoms that thyroid patients report is itching. Some of this may be caused by dryness, but often a condition known as *dermatographism* may play a role in the itching. Simply stated, skin trauma such as scratching or even a hot shower produces hives that itch (Figure 63). This troublesome symptom can be helped by substituting lukewarm baths for hot showers and avoiding substances that irritate the skin (wool is a common culprit).

CHAPTER TEN

Thyroid Lumps and Tumors

Thyroid lumps or nodules are common, and a careful thyroid examination will reveal thyroid lumps larger than a centimeter (⅖ inch) in diameter in 4 percent of the population. Furthermore, autopsy studies in which the entire gland has been carefully examined have shown that small thyroid nodules are, in fact, much more common than that and can be found in more than half of the population.

Fortunately, most of these nodules are harmless and require no treatment. Although cancer does occur, it is an extremely rare condition. The United States Public Health Service reports that in one year only 25 people per *million* in the population will be found to have a cancer in the thyroid gland. Therefore, if you or your physician have found a lump in your throat (Figure 22), don't panic. Although it is important that the nodule be evaluated, it is unlikely to be a cancer. It is far more likely to be benign (harmless).

EVALUATING A THYROID NODULE*

Your physician will take a careful medical history, examine your neck, and perform some laboratory tests to gain the information needed to decide if your thyroid lump should be surgically removed.

*See also Tables 2 and 3, on page 000 in this chapter.

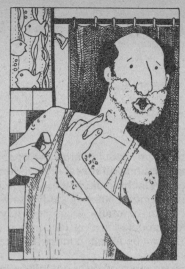

Figure 22 If you find a lump in your neck, see your doctor.

By talking with you about your medical history, your physician can get a good idea of whether your nodule is likely to be benign or cancerous. For example, a lump is more likely to be benign if you are an adult woman who has symptoms of an overactive or underactive thyroid, or who has relatives with benign conditions such as chronic lymphocytic thyroiditis or a goiter. On the other hand, if you are a child, or an adolescent, or a male, or if you had x-ray treatments to the thyroid region sometime in the past, chances are greater that the lump is a cancer. There is also a greater likelihood of cancer if you have noticed rapid enlargement of the nodule or a change in your voice, hoarseness, or trouble in swallowing (suggesting that a cancer is pressing against nearby parts of your neck).

During a physical examination, your physician will feel your thyroid gland. Benign nodules tend to be soft and fleshy, and are not associated with enlargement of nearby lymph glands. The rest of the thyroid also may feel abnormal. It is particularly reassuring if more than one nodule can be felt within the thyroid, since this is an indication of a generalized thyroid disease, such as a nodular goiter. On the other hand, if your doctor feels a single, hard, fixed lump in an otherwise apparently normal gland, that nodule is more likely to contain cancer. The likelihood of cancer increases if the lump seems "fixed" to nearby structures within your neck or if it is associated with swelling of nearby lymph glands.

After your physician has examined your neck, tests will probably be recommended depending on the findings in your examination. Fortunately, the testing techniques available today usually make it possible to distinguish harmless lumps that can be left alone or treated medically from cancerous tumors that must be removed.

Blood tests that reveal high or low thyroid hormone levels or the presence of antithyroid antibodies (suggesting the presence of chronic lymphocytic thyroiditis) help to indicate that a lump is probably harmless. But a radioiodine thyroid scan is far more useful, for it provides evidence of the way the nodule itself is functioning.

In order to have a thyroid scan made, you will be given a small amount of radioiodine* to swallow in a capsule or in a small amount of water. Twenty-four hours later a scan picture is made that creates an image of your entire thyroid gland (Figure 23). The position of your nodule can be located on the scan, making it possible to compare the function of the nodule with that of the surrounding thyroid tissue. In addition, the scan provides helpful information about the function of the rest of your thyroid, sometimes showing the presence of other

*We have found that a radidoactive *iodine* scan is more helpful in evaluating thyroid lumps than a scan done with radioactive *technetium* (see Chapter 2). At the Massachusetts General Hospital we have *never* seen a cancerous nodule that concentrated radioiodine normally in a thyroid scan. In contrast, an occasional thyroid cancer will concentrate technitium and give the misleading impression that the nodule is functioning and therefore harmless.

abnormal areas elsewhere in the gland (Figure 26). Such a scan pattern suggests the presence of several nodules, a harmless condition known as a multinodular goiter.

In a general way, you can think of thyroid nodules as *hot* (functional) or *cold* (nonfunctional). A *hot* nodule is one that concentrates radioiodine equal to or more than the surrounding thyroid tissue. Occasionally, the rest of the thyroid is not even visible on the scan because the hot nodule is making so much thyroid hormone that the function of the rest of the thyroid gland is suppressed

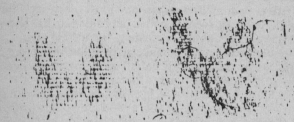

Figure 23 An artist's rendering of a normal thyroid scan.

Figure 26 A multinodular goiter has several "hot" and "cold" areas, which cause the pattern to appear "patchy." (An artist's rendering)

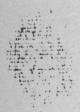
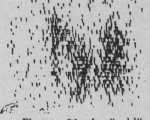

Figure 25 A "hot" thyroid nodule is the part of this thyroid that took up radioiodine. (An artist's rendering)

Figure 24 A "cold" nodule does not take up radioiodine and appears as a "hole" in an otherwise normal thyroid scan. (An artist's rendering)

(Figure 25). In our experience, hot nodules are *never* malignant.

A nodule that concentrates radioiodine poorly or not at all is termed *cold* (Figure 24). Although all cancers are cold, most benign tumors and cysts are also cold. In fact, only about 10 percent of solitary cold nodules prove to be malignant. However, the *presence of a cold nodule is always an indication for further evaluation.* Moreover, it is more likely to contain cancer if the radioiodine scan shows it to be the only inactive area in an otherwise normal-appearing thyroid gland.

FURTHER MANAGEMENT OF THYROID NODULES

If you have a hot nodule, you probably do not need any treatment. Follow-up is important because such a nodule can, in time, produce too much thyroid hormone. If this occurs, treatment is usually recommended in order to control symptoms of hyperthyroidism (see Chapter 5).

If your nodule is *cold* on scan, however, it must be determined whether the lump is nonfunctional because it contains cancer, because it is a fluid-filled cyst, or because it is simply one of the harmless types of solid thyroid tumors.

At this point, your physician's choice of tests may depend on what tests are possible in the office or hospital where you are being examined. In many hospitals it is possible to do an *ultrasound test*, a painless procedure that utilizes sound waves much as radar would to create a picture of the thyroid gland. Cysts appear to be dark or "echo-free" areas, quite different from the way solid tumors look (Figure 68). However, a drawback of the ultrasound test is that it cannot tell with certainty whether a solid tumor is harmless or cancerous. Therefore, most solid cold nodules will need to be either biopsied or removed in a thyroid operation.

If you have several hot and/or cold nodules in your thyroid, you probably have the very common condition known as *multinodular goiter* (see Chapter 3). These goiters rarely contain cancer. They are made up of hot and cold nodules that produce a characteristic "patchy" uptake of radioiodine throughout the gland in a thyroid scan picture (Figure 26). If that is your situation, or if you have a single nodule that is too small to biopsy, or one that is located in a part of your thyroid that cannot be simply biopsied, your physician may choose to observe the nodule for a few months. During the period of observation you may be treated with thyroid hormone in pill form, either to try to shrink the nodule or to shrink the surrounding tissue and thus make the nodule easier to feel. Thyroid hormone pills are often used in this way. They act by "turning off" your pituitary gland's production of thyroid stimulating hormone. The lack of stimulation by TSH causes many (but not all) benign nodules and all normal thyroid tissue to decrease in size. In fact, if your nodule does get smaller during treatment with thyroid hormone pills, that is an indication to your physician that your nodule is benign.

During treatment with thyroid hormone, your physician will probably ask you to return periodically for evaluation. One reason for checkups is to be sure that you are not developing hyperthyroidism, which could happen if the amount of thyroid hormone produced by the overactive parts of your thyroid gland plus the amount of hormone in your thyroid pills adds up to more than your body should have. If so, your doctor will probably lower your dose of thyroid and reexamine you at a later date.*

---

*As we say in Chapter 5, if you have a multinodular goiter, you may also become hyperthyroid if you increase your iodine intake abruptly. This might happen if you begin to eat kelp or start to take an iodine-containing medication. Therefore, if you have a multinodular goiter, read labels of any medications or over-the-counter health remedies to be sure they do not contain iodine. If you have a question about this, consult your physician.

†A photographic and written account of a thyroid biopsy can be found at the end of this chapter.

THYROID BIOPSY†

Often blood tests, thyroid scan, and ultrasound tests do not enable a physician to tell whether a nodule is benign or malignant. In that case, a thyroid *biopsy* may be advised.

The term *biopsy* refers to either of two procedures that are performed to get a sample of thyroid tissue for examination under a microscope. To perform the test, your physician will numb the skin of your neck with a local anesthetic and will then insert a needle into your thyroid nodule, either to remove fluid (proving it to be a cyst) or to get a small sample of tissue for microscopic examination. In a *fine needle aspiration*, small numbers of thyroid cells are sucked out of the thyroid gland through a small needle attached to a syringe. In contrast, in a *cutting needle biopsy*, use of a larger hollow needle permits the removal of a core of thyroid tissue for examination. These procedures, both in common use today, are safe in experienced hands and are normally carried out in a physician's office. Individual physicians generally prefer the technique with which they have had most experience and which gives them the most reliable results.

Most physicians currently perform the fine-needle aspiration biopsy because it is technically easier. However, the results of the fine-needle biopsy tend to be less definitive than the cutting-needle biopsy. Because of this problem, some tests will be inconclusive. In such instances, your physician will probably recommend one of three courses of action: an operation to remove the nodule, rebiopsy with a fine or cutting needle, or a period of observation of the nodule while you take thyroid hormone treatment, followed by a reexamination of you and your nodule a few weeks or months later.

On the other hand, your physician may recommend surgical removal of the nodule instead of a biopsy. This will provide an accurate diagnosis and will, of course, be a definitive form of treatment as well.

IF THE NODULE PROVES CANCEROUS ... WHAT THEN?

Even in those rare instances when a cold nodule proves to be a thyroid cancer, it should not necessarily be a cause for alarm. Typically, thyroid cancer grows slowly and often can be completely removed surgically. In those instances when the tumor cannot be entirely removed, it usually responds to treatment with thyroid hormone and radioactive iodine, occasionally supplemented with x-ray treatment and chemotherapy.

If it seems possible that your cancer has spread, your physician may want to measure the level of a substance known as *thyroglobulin* in a sample of your blood. Thyroglobulin is a large protein in which thyroid hormones are normally stored in your thyroid. The amount of thyroglobulin in your blood is normally small, but it may increase if you have a thyroid cancer that has spread from your thyroid to other body tissues. Thus, it is possible to use a measurement of the thyroglobulin level in a blood test to help decide if cancer has spread, or if cancer once thought cured has recurred.

There are several types of thyroid cancer. They include *follicular*, *papillary*, and *Hürthle cell* cancers. *Anaplastic* cancer is a serious, rapidly spreading type of tumor that is made up of immature (undifferentiated) thyroid cells. Recommended treatment will depend on the type and extent of tumor that is present. Whatever the treatment, most patients will be placed on lifelong therapy with thyroid hormone tablets.* Just as in the

---

*As we have emphasized elsewhere, the only thyroid hormone preparations we use for such treatment are Levothroid and Synthroid. In Canada, in addition to Synthroid, Eltroxin is also reliable. Generic thyroxine prescriptions are not recommended because the tablets vary too much in potency.

case of benign nodules and normal thyroid tissue, many forms of thyroid cancer are dependent on TSH for growth. Hence, thyroid hormone is administered in an effort to "suppress" the secretion of TSH from the pituitary, and thereby prevent growth of the thyroid cancer. With most thyroid cancer, complete cure is common, and the outlook with treatment is excellent.

About 10 percent of thyroid cancers are somewhat unusual tumors known as *medullary carcinomas*. These tumors may be discovered as a single hard lump in the neck like other forms of thyroid cancer. In such cases, they should be evaluated like other thyroid nodules, and often they can be successfully treated by surgical removal.

In some patients, however, these tumors develop as part of an inherited disorder, and in such individuals more than one medullary cancer can usually be found within the thyroid gland. Patients with this condition may also develop tumors of the adrenal glands (which can cause high blood pressure) and parathyroid glands (which can raise the blood calcium level). In some patients nerve tumors (neuromas) may also appear.

Medullary thyroid cancer cells produce a protein known as *calcitonin*, which can be detected by a blood test. Calcitonin measurements are helpful in several ways. First, the presence of calcitonin in the blood tells us what kind of thyroid tumor the patient has. Second, if it is still present in the patient's blood after thyroid surgery has been completed, it means that not all of the tumor has been removed and that more tumor treatment is needed. Finally, if a patient has the inherited type of medullary thyroid cancer, physicians can use calcitonin blood tests to find out which relatives have the same condition before the tumor has fully developed. This is vitally important, for those relatives who have the best opportunity to be cured of this cancer are those in whom evidence of the tumor is found in childhood, before spread of the tumor cells from the thyroid has occurred.

Obviously, medullary thyroid carcinoma is a tumor with many characteristics that make it different from other types of cancer. Therefore, if you or a member of your family has this type of thyroid problem it is very important that you find out from your physician whether other family members should also be tested for evidence of this disorder.

In summary, physicians have at their disposal ways to accurately diagnose the cause of a thyroid nodule. In most instances, tests will show that the nodule is harmless, and surgery unnecessary. When studies suggest that cancer is likely to be present in a thyroid nodule, surgery alone may be curative, though other forms of treatment are available when needed.

Table 2 is a comparison of clues that may be present and suggest that a particular nodule is either benign or malignant. It must be realized that these characteristics are only *indicators*—not *proof*—of the nature of the lump. Therefore, under most circumstances your physician will perform thyroid tests (Table 3).

A THYROID BIOPSY

by S. S.

The doctor's quiet and calm manner set the tone for the procedure. First, he examined my neck with his fingers. This didn't hurt at all. Then he drew a picture on paper showing me where my thyroid lump was in my thyroid gland. He explained what he was going to do, and why it was important to do it.

We then walked into his examining room. I unbuttoned the top three or four buttons on my shirt, and lay on my back on his examining table. The nurse put pillows under my shoulders so that my head hung back. It felt like I was upside down. This position exposed my neck area, which was washed with alcohol. Doctor Wang told me he was going to inject Novocain into my

TABLE 2

Characteristics of Cancerous and Benign Thyroid Nodules
(History and Physical Examination)

The likelihood that a nodule is a cancer is increased if:

The likelihood that a nodule is benign is increased if:

HISTORY

the patient is a child or adolescent.

the patient is male.

the patient has had x-ray treatment to the head, neck, or chest in childhood.

the patient has noticed rapid enlargement of the nodule.

the patient has noticed a change in voice, hoarseness, or trouble in swallowing, suggesting compression of nearby neck structures.

the patient is an adult.

the patient is female.

the patient has symptoms of an overactive or underactive thyroid.

the patient has a strong family history of benign thyroid diseases such as chronic lymphocytic thyroiditis or multinodular goiter.

PHYSICAL EXAMINATION

a single lump is felt in the thyroid.

the lump is "fixed" (attached) to the tissues around it.

the nearby neck lymph glands are enlarged.

the rest of the thyroid feels normal.

more than one lump is felt in the thyroid.

no lymph node enlargement can be found.

the rest of the thyroid feels abnormal (firm, enlarged, irregular, etc).

TABLE 3

Characteristics of Cancerous and Benign
Thyroid Nodules
(Thyroid Tests)

	The likelihood that a nodule is a cancer is increased if:	*The likelihood that a nodule is benign is increased if:*
Thyroid hormone blood level	is normal.	is high or low (but often will be normal).
Antithyroid antibody in blood	is absent.	is present.
Radioiodine scan	shows that lump is "cold" or "cool" concentrating radioiodine poorly.	shows that lump concentrates radioiodine.
Thyroid ultrasound	shows solid tumor.	shows a cyst (but often benign tumors will be solid).
Thyroid aspiration or needle biopsy	reveals cancer cells.	reveals cyst fluid or benign tissue cells.

neck. The needle felt like a pin prick or a mosquito bite.

After a few minutes the Novocain had numbed my neck, and Doctor Wang proceeded with the biopsy itself. This meant that he put a needle through the numb skin on my neck into my thyroid lump. The only feeling on my neck during the procedure was slight pressure. There was absolutely no pain or discomfort. Toward the end I felt a little dizzy and clammy, probably due to my nervousness and to the fact that my head was in an upside down position. The doctor kept explaining and talking to me during the whole procedure so that I always knew what was going on and never felt afraid.

After the biopsy was over, I held a gauze pad against the place on my neck where the biopsy had been done. The pillow under my shoulders was removed, and I was asked to lie quietly for about ten minutes. During this time all my dizziness went away. Soon the nurse put a small Band-Aid on the biopsy place on my neck. Then I got up and walked into Dr. Wang's outer office, where I waited for a few more minutes. Then I left his office, drove home, and ate supper. There was no pain, discomfort, or dizziness.

Later that night I noticed a sore feeling as if I had a slight bruise on my neck. There was also slight swelling where the biopsy had been done. However, there was no real pain or serious discomfort.

A THYROID NODULE DISCOVERED, TESTED, AND REMOVED

by H. J.

During a physical examination, my doctor told me he thought he felt a lump or "nodule" in my thyroid gland. Because of this he took a blood sample to measure my thyroid hormone level and ordered a thyroid scan. My blood test was normal, but the scan, which was made using a small dose of radioactive iodine that I had swallowed the day before, showed that there was a nodule as suspected, and that it was not "functioning." That means it did not take up iodine as the rest of the thyroid gland did, appearing instead like an empty hole in the scan picture (see Figure 24).

Thet next step was a thyroid biopsy. This was performed by a surgeon and was done to learn what kind of thyroid tissue was in the nodule, and thus determine whether it had to be removed in an operation.

I was relieved to discover that a biopsy was not much more difficult or painful for me than having a blood sample taken. The surgeon asked me to loosen a few buttons of my shirt and lie on my back with my neck extended over a bunched-up pillow to better expose the front of my neck where the thyroid is located. After cleaning my neck with alcohol he numbed the skin with a local anesthetic. After the skin was numb he made a tiny incision about ⅛ inch long in the skin. Through this "hole" he inserted a needle into the thyroid nodule, and through the needle he was able to obtain the biopsy specimen—a small cylinder of tissue. During the biopsy I felt a pressure sensation in my neck but no pain. I also had an urge to cough (but suppressed it) when the surgeon pressed on my windpipe. Afterward, I held a cotton bandage on the biopsy site for about five minutes. Then my "wound" was covered with a small Band-Aid. I got up without any ill effects and went home to await the report of the biopsy.

After examining the biopsy specimen, my physicians agreed that an operation was indicated. The surgeon told me about the operation that he planned to do—a "partial thyroidectomy." This meant that only the left lobe of the thyroid, which contained the nodule, was to be removed. I was told that more extensive surgery might be required if the examination during surgery revealed the presence of more widespread disease than expected. I learned that I would be admitted the day before surgery for a physical examination and tests of my general health. I was told that I could expect a sore throat for several days after surgery, but that I would be able to eat breakfast the morning after surgery. I was to plan to take 2 to 3 weeks off work after surgery because I would feel tired.

A week later I was admitted to the hospital. In the afternoon, routine preoperative tests were performed, including a chest x-ray, an electrocardiogram, and blood and urine tests. That evening, an anesthesiologist came to my room and told me a little about what would happen. He said that I could not eat or drink after midnight. If I wanted, I could get an injection to relax me on the morning of surgery before being taken to the operating room. He told me that an "IV" would be put in my arm through which I would be given an injection to put me to sleep. After I was asleep, a plastic tube would be inserted through my mouth into my windpipe in order to give me oxygen and anesthetic gases during the operation. He said that I would feel groggy for a few hours after I woke up and that I might be nauseated.

Things went pretty much as everyone had said. I slept remarkably well the night before surgery, although I was a little anxious. I was wide awake and hungry the morning of surgery (although of course I couldn't have anything to eat). A surgical orderly dressed in a "scrub suit," hair net, and mask came into my room with a stretcher for me to lie on. He took me through various corridors to the operating room area, and then parked my stretcher in a little cubicle outside the room in which my operation would take place. Soon an operating room nurse and a nurse-anesthetist came to my side. They asked me my name and whether I had any allergies, as well as a few of the other questions I had been asked before, just to make sure everything was in order. Finally, the nurse-anesthetist started the IV in my arm. Shortly thereafter I spotted my surgeon standing nearby. After speaking briefly with my surgeon and hearing some encouraging words from the people around me, I was given an intravenous injection of morphine that made my whole body tingle and began to make me drowsy. At this point I was wheeled into the operating room itself. I was still awake and set about arranging myself on the operating table, but the masked faces of the people around me gradually drifted out of sight as sodium pentothal was injected into my IV and I fell asleep.

When I awoke, I was lying on a bed in the recovery room. Here I was to spend the next few hours to be sure that there were no complications from the operation following surgery. I had a very sore throat and it was hard for me to swallow. I felt very drugged. I could open my eyes for about five seconds, recognize people, read the clock on the wall, even talk, but then I would drift back to sleep. I did not need any pain medication during this time.

After about four hours, I was taken back to my hospital room where I drifted in and out of sleep until about 9 P.M. Then, about eight hours after surgery and still with a sore throat and difficulty in swallowing, I woke up for several hours, although I felt very weak. I was able to walk to the bathroom with assistance, although it took several attempts before I was able to empty my obviously full bladder—an effect of the anesthetic drugs. I was able to sip ginger ale through a straw although every swallow hurt. I slept on and off throughout the night, and I refused pain medication because the grogginess and nausea from the drugs seemed worse than the sore throat from surgery.

I was considerably more awake the next morning and managed to swallow a soft breakfast. My IV came out (thank goodness—my hand was hurting). Then a small rubber drain in my neck was removed, and a suture was tied where it had been (all painless).

During the rest of my hospital stay my throat gradually became less and less sore. On the fifth day my stitches were removed and I went home. I felt weak and tired easily for about a week but had recovered full strength by two weeks after surgery. The swelling around the site of surgery and the mild tenderness over the left side of my neck (where the nodule and thyroid lobe were removed) also resolved during that time.

CHAPTER ELEVEN

Thyroid Trouble in Children

If your child's thyroid is not working properly, it is likely to have different effects than it would if you had the same problem. This is because your child is growing and developing, and growth and development can be changed by a thyroid that is either overactive (hyperthyroid) or underactive (hypothyroid).

In addition, thyroid trouble can be more difficult to recognize in a child than in an adult. Children are less likely to complain of feeling sick or to ask for help. They do not know what "normal" is, so even older children may simply accept the emotional and physical symptoms of a thyroid problem as "normal" for them. Therefore, it's usually up to someone else to recognize thyroid diseases when they occur in children. Indeed, an increase in irritability or hyperactivity noticed by a parent, friend, or teacher, or a change in growth rate noted by a parent or pediatrician may be the clue that leads to the discovery of a thyroid problem in a child.

Finally, since some thyroid disorders are inherited—passed on from one generation to the next—we would like to stress one very important point: If someone in the family has thyroid trouble now or has had a thyroid problem in the past, be sure to tell the child's physician about it. If it is the type of thyroid trouble that can be inherited, you will have alerted the physician to be watchful for that problem in the child.

GOITER IN CHILDHOOD

Any time the thyroid grows larger than normal, it is called a *goiter*. A goiter may appear at any age but is especially common in girls about the time their menstrual cycles begin.

If your child develops a goiter, it is possible that he or she is still healthy and no important thyroid problem exists. On the other hand, most goiters that appear in children over six years of age are caused by low-grade inflammation* of the thyroid gland known as *chronic lymphocytic thyroiditis* or *Hashimoto's disease*.† In adults, this condition is a common cause of thyroid failure (see Chapter 7). Occasionally, a goiter may be the first sign of some other thyroid problem: Your child's thyroid may be overactive, or it may be enlarged due to inflammation associated with a viral infection.

Therefore, if you notice a goiter in your child, you should take the child to a physician for a checkup. By examining the child and obtaining a blood test, the doctor can tell if the thyroid gland is overactive or underactive. Either of these thyroid conditions may interfere with a child's growth and development, but treating them will correct the thyroid hormone level and restore the growth pattern to normal.

Even if the results of the examination and the thyroid tests in a child with a goiter are normal, that does not mean necessarily that the goiter can be forgotten. Rather, the physician will probably reexamine and retest your child at a later time to be sure a change in thyroid function has not occurred.

Rarely, a child's neck will have a swelling that appears to be a generalized enlargement of the entire thyroid

---

*Inflammation in this context does not mean an infection is present.

†This type of thyroiditis is so named in honor of the Japanese physician who described it.

gland but may actually be caused by an enlarged over-
lying fat pad or by growth of one or more lumps or nodules in the thyroid. The enlarged fat pad, which can be
recognized by the fact that it does not move up and
down with the Adam's apple when the child swallows, is
of no significance. In the case of nodules, however, medical evaluation, as outlined later in this chapter, is very
important and should be carried out promptly. Although
most nodules prove to be harmless cysts or tumors, occasionally they contain thyroid cancer or reflect a
change of thyroid function. Such conditions can and
should be treated.

THE OVERACTIVE THYROID
IN CHILDHOOD

One of the best understood forms of thyroid trouble in
children is the increased thyroid activity that affects
some newborn babies and is known as *neonatal hyp-
perthyroidism*. This condition is rare,* occurring only in
infants born of mothers with a hyperthyroid condition. It
is due to the passage of chemical substances called *thyroid stimulators* from the mother's blood across the placenta to her unborn baby. When these substances get
into the baby's blood stream, they may cause the baby's
thyroid to make too much thyroid hormone.

Fortunately, this type of hyperthyroidism in a newborn baby lasts only as long as the mother's thyroid stimulators remain in the baby's blood stream, usually from
three to twelve weeks. Moreover, the condition is
usually mild, since most women who have an overactive
thyroid do not have very high blood levels of the thyroid
stimulators. Occasionally, a mother will have such high

*Only about 100 such infants have been described so far in the medical
literature, and only one of every 70 babies born to mothers who are hyperthyroid during pregnancy develop this condition.

levels of the stimulators that her baby will be born with prominent eyes, irritability, flushing of the skin, and a fast pulse—all characteristics of an overactive thyroid at any age. In addition, such babies are long and scrawny and may have tremendous appetites but not gain weight. A goiter is common but may not be obvious at birth.

In its mildest form, this disease may require no treatment and will subside by itself in time. However, if the baby is seriously ill, treatment with iodine and an antithyroid drug such as propylthiouracil may be required to control the overactive thyroid gland. If more rapid control of symptoms is required, treatment with a *beta adrenergic blocking drug* like atenolol or propranolol may be helpful. The drug works by blocking the action of the high thyroid hormone levels on the baby's body. Thyroid surgery is rarely if ever needed, even if the baby has a very large thyroid, for treatment with iodine usually causes the gland to shrink rapidly in size. This is fortunate, since a thyroid operation would be extremely difficult in so tiny a patient. Treatment can usually be discontinued in a few weeks, for the mother's thyroid stimulators soon disappear from the baby's blood stream.

Even though this condition is extremely rare, a pregnant woman who has hyperthyroidism or who has been hyperthyroid in the past* should alert the obstetrician about her thyroid problem *during the pregnancy* so that her doctor will be prepared to look for a thyroid abnormality in the baby.

Hyperthroidism that occurs in children after the newborn period is very much like hyperthyroidism in adults. However, children generally do not complain of such things as having too much energy or feeling nervous, so it may be hard to tell if your child is sick with an overactive thyroid, even though you may be exhausted by a

---

*Such a woman may have thyroid stimulators in her blood that cannot make *her* hyperthyroid if her thyroid has been removed or treated yet can go across the placenta and make her unborn baby hyperthyroid.

hyperactive and restless child who never seems to need a nap (Figure 27). Quite often the *only* clue that a problem exists will be a sudden growth spurt that makes a child with an overactive thyroid suddenly grow taller. A pediatrician who keeps careful records of the child's body measurements may notice such a change, but more often parents become aware of a sudden increase in growth when their child rapidly outgrows new clothes.

There are other clues by which we can recognize hyperthyroidism. Virtually all hyperthyroid children have a goiter and prominent eyes. Other common signs of thyroid overactivity include a rapid pulse, nervousness, increased sweating, and a dislike for hot weather. Parents may notice a deterioration of school perform-

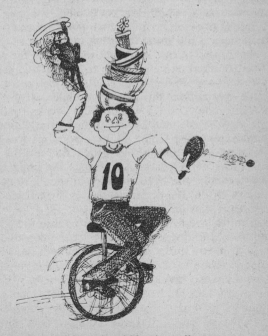

Figure 21   A hyperthyroid child has boundless energy.

ance, and the teacher may report that the child doesn't pay attention in class. Rapid growth of fingernails may lead to accumulation of dirt under irregular nail margins. Shaky hands may cause clumsiness and poor handwriting, while weak shoulder and thigh muscles may be apparent in play or sports. Emotional disturbances may be seen, and parents commonly note that even a gentle reprimand brings forth a flood of tears.

If you suspect that your child has an overactive thyroid, he or she should be examined by a physician. Usually, a blood sample will be obtained for measurement of the child's thyroid hormone level. If the diagnosis is confirmed, the doctor may be able to start treatment at once. Adults suspected of having this condition usually are tested with a radioactive thyroid uptake and scan, which are performed to prove that the thyroid is overactive and to gain more information about the thyroid gland itself. These tests are not always done in children in whom the diagnosis is clear; the physician wants to avoid exposing them to radioactive substances that may be more harmful to children than to adults.

An overactive thyroid in a child usually can be brought under control within a few weeks by treatment with one of the antithyroid drugs: propylthiouracil or methimazole (Tapazole). Many physicians will continue treatment with antithyroid drugs for several months, sometimes even years. As long as the child takes the drugs reliably, the hyperthyroidism should remain under control. Often, the disease subsides by itself and a *spontaneous remission* occurs.

If this is the form of treatment chosen for your child, you should know something about the possible side effects from the drugs. Some children will develop an allergic reaction to the medications, usually manifested as fever, itching, hives, or a red skin rash. Very rarely, these antithyroid drugs may produce a more serious problem, lowering or even causing the complete disappearance of certain of the child's white blood cells (neutrophils), which help to protect the child from infections.* Therefore, if your child is taking one of these drugs and develops fever, itching, hives, a skin rash, or evidence of an infection (such as sore throat, sore mouth, or fever), the child should stop taking the drug† and the physician should be notified at once. If the doctor finds that your child is allergic to the antithyroid drug, another form of treatment will be recommended. On the other hand, if the problem is a fever or infection, the child may be able to continue drug treatment even while the infection is being treated, provided the neutrophil count is normal.

Fortunately, antithyroid drugs do not usually cause serious problems, and most children can take them safely. But if reactions occur, or if the hyperthyroidism cannot be properly controlled by these medications, or if the thyroid remains very large and unsightly, the doctor may recommend that much of the child's thyroid gland be removed surgically. Once the thyroid tissue is removed, the source of the excessive amounts of thyroid hormone is gone and the child should be cured. Indeed, thyroid surgery is usually safe and effective if the surgeon is well-trained and experienced in thyroid surgery in children. Unfortunately, this kind of surgery can be difficult, carrying with it the risk of damage to structures in the neck near the thyroid gland (Figure 28). A few children who are operated upon for hyperthyroidism will have surgical injury to the nerve supplying their vocal cords. Accidental removal of or damage to the nearby parathyroid glands may also occur. The former may cause a change in voice or permanent hoarseness, while the latter may produce a calcium imbalance for which the child may need to take medication for the rest of his

*This most serious complication of drug therapy, known as "agranulocytosis," happens to only about one child in every three hundred who take propylthiouracil or methimazole. Yet the seriousness of this possible complication makes us give it special attention.

†Some physicians prefer to see the child before the drug is stopped to be sure that another condition (such as measles or poison ivy) is not being mistaken for a drug rash.

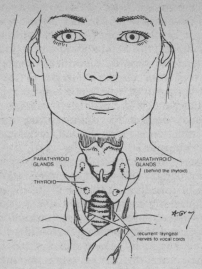

Figure 28 Normal location of the parathyroid glands and recurrent laryngeal nerves.

or her life. In addition, a surgical scar will result, though it usually fades and becomes less noticeable with the passage of time.

In view of such potentially serious complications from drug and surgical treatments for hyperthyroidism in children, it would seem that physicians would choose instead to control the thyroid as we usually do in adults, by destroying some of the thyroid with radioactive iodine. Indeed, this treatment is as effective as surgical removal of the thyroid and carries no risk of damage to the vocal cord nerves or parathyroid glands. However, although it is clear that no serious complications from radioactive iodine treatment have been observed in more than forty years' experience in treating adults, physicians are aware that very young children's thyroid glands may be sensitive to the effects of radiation and they may be more likely to develop thyroid tumors and other complications in the years following such treatment. Also, in contrast to adults, children have more years ahead of them in which to develop complications from radiation. Fortunately, at this time there is no evidence that children who have been treated with radioiodine have developed any specific problems.

Radioactive iodine is an effective means of controlling hyperthyroidism in a child, and it may prove to be as safe in children as in adults. For the time being, however, most physicians do not routinely use this treatment for children. Instead, we reserve radioiodine for use in children who are allergic to antithyroid drugs or whose hyperthyroidism cannot be controlled by such drugs, and in whom thyroid surgery is not advisable for some reason. You and your physician should discuss the alternatives of treatmenet of your child's condition carefully in an effort to understand the particular circumstances that lead to a recommendation of a specific plan of treatment.

Hyperthyroidism of the type that commonly occurs among children is a lifelong disease. It may recur at any time, and in some cases the gland may fail, resulting in hypothyroidism. Children treated surgically or with radioiodine are particulary apt to develop hypothyroidism. For these reasons, any hyperthyroid child should remain under the guidance of a physician indefinitely. If the thyroid does fail, hypothyroidism can be treated easily with thyroid hormone replacement tablets once a day.

THE UNDERACTIVE THYROID IN CHILDHOOD

In our country one in every four to five thousand babies is born with hypothyroidism. Here, as in most developed countries, hypothyroidism in the newborn usually is due to an absent or abnormally located and poorly functioning thyroid gland. Hypothyroidism can be seen also in infants born to mothers who took antithyroid drugs or iodine during pregnancy, either of which can pass from the mother to her baby and affect the baby's thyroid. Finally, 10 percent of the time hypothyroidism is due to one of several known inherited disorders in which the thyroid makes too little thyroid hormone as a result of a defect in the hormone manufacturing process.

Hypothyroidism is even more common in some remote, often mountainous, areas of the world where there is insufficient iodine in the diet. Such iodine-deficient infants may suffer mental and physical damage from which they cannot recover even if they are eventually treated adequately with thyroid hormone. Iodine deficiency is not a problem in the United States because our salt is iodized and iodine has been added to other foods as well.

If you have a baby born with an underactive thyroid, the baby may seem normal to you and even to the doctor who checks the infant after birth. In the next hours and days you may notice that the baby's skin has a yellowish color due to newborn *jaundice*, which clears slowly in hypothyroid babies. It is only in the following days and weeks that the infant becomes sluggish, sleepy, and develops the hoarse cry, stuffy nose, and puffy face and body typical of the kind of hypothyroidism known as *cretinism*. But by then your baby would be at home and you might not realize at first that he or she was seriously sick. The problem is that if such a baby is not treated with thyroid hormone as soon as possible after birth, permanent brain damage and mental retardation may occur.

Fortunately, if hypothyroidism due to any cause is discovered early and treated appropriately, permanent damage to the child usually can be avoided. However, IT MUST BE DIAGNOSED AS EARLY AS POSSIBLE— PREFERABLY WITH BLOOD TESTS DONE AT BIRTH. Moreover, since permanent brain damage *can* be prevented with early treatment,* many physicians throughout most of North America, as well as in many other parts of the world, are now screening *all* newborn babies for hypothyroidism by means of tests done on blood obtained by heel prick or from the umbilical cord.

Infant thyroid screening is encouragingly successful and should be performed throughout the world, and now all babies are screened throughout the United States and Canada.

Finally, in addition to being certain your baby will have thyroid tests done immediately after birth, you *must* read carefully labels of all medicines you take during pregnancy, and ascertain that they do not contain large quantities of iodine or other substances known to affect the baby. Iodized table salt poses no problem, but health foods like kelp and some medications (for example, certain cough syrups) contain large amounts of iodine. If they are taken in large quantities over a long period, they may cause not only thyroid deficiency, but also goiter in your baby. Obviously, during pregnancy, antithyroid drugs should be used in only the lowest possible dose and under the close supervision of a physician, and radioactive iodine (which might damage the baby's thyroid) should NEVER be given to a pregnant woman for any reason.

HYPOTHYROIDISM IN LATER CHILDHOOD

If your child's thyroid fails after the child is six years old, the thyroid is probably affected by a low-grade inflammation* known as *chronic lymphocytic thyroiditis*.

---

*The kind of inflammation present in chronic lymphocytic thyroiditis is not associated with infection.

*Most pediatricians feel that such children must be treated with thyroid hormone before they are three months old if serious brain damage is to be prevented.

The first sign that such a problem exists is often a painless swelling in the front of the neck caused by the enlarged thyroid. Fortunately, this slight enlargement of the thyroid is usually enough to alert the pediatrician or the parents to the fact that thyroid disease is present. Since this type of thyroiditis can damage thyroid tissue and thus decrease thyroid function, symptoms and signs of hypothyroidism may follow. However, such a child may seem perfectly healthy, and the *only* evidence that the thyroid is failing may be a slowing of the growth rate. In such a case, the pediatrician may be the first to suspect hypothyroidism when the child's growth rate slows and fails to keep up with the past growth pattern. Parents may have noticed symptoms of hypothyroidism long before that, including sluggishness (Figure 29), pallor, dry and itchy skin, increased sensitivity to cold, and constipation. At the same time, surprisingly, schoolwork may improve. Once hypothyroidism is suspected, the physician usually has no trouble in confirming the diagnosis, for a blood test will reveal a low thyroid hormone level as well as an elevated level of the pituitary thyroid stimulating hormone described in detail in Chapters 6 and 7. Treatment of the hypothyroidism with thyroid hormone

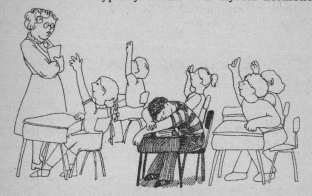

Figure 29 A hypothyroid child may be less active than normal during the day.

should correct the symptoms and signs of the condition, with rapid improvement in energy and mental function, followed by a return to normal of the growth pattern. Do not be surprised if schoolwork suffers temporarily as the treated child becomes more aware of the environment and more involved in outside activities.

PAINFUL SWELLING OF THE THYROID (SUBACUTE THYROIDITIS)

Occasionally, a week or two after a viral infection (often a typical sore throat) an older child may begin to complain of an unusual type of sore throat. In such an illness, the discomfort may be coming from a painfully swollen thyroid gland in the front of the neck. Your child may have a fever, aches, and pains and may be sick enough to stay in bed, but it is the tender goiter that suggests thyroid inflammation is present—not just a "common cold."

Blood tests usually will prove that your child's swollen thyroid is inflamed. If there is any doubt, the pediatrician may do a radioactive thyroid uptake test, which should show no activity at all in the inflamed thyroid gland. Typical treatment is with aspirin alone, and rapid improvement usually is apparent within a day or two.

On rare occasions when the condition is severe, there may be an early period of perhaps three to four weeks during which your child may develop symptoms of hyperthyroidism due to large amounts of thyroid hormone that have leaked out of the inflamed gland. This may be followed by another three to four weeks during which your child may be sluggish from low thyroid levels until the exhausted gland begins to work again. If either of these phases is severe, the physician can prescribe medications to control symptoms, correct the thyroid hormone level, and make the child feel better. Once the disease has run its course, the child should recover completely and remain healthy.

THYROID NODULES

Thyroid nodules (lumps) that appear in childhood are usually due to thyroid inflammation (thyroiditis), benign (harmless) tumors, or thyroid cysts. Fortunately, thyroid nodules containing cancer are rare in children. If your child develops a thyroid cancer, it probably will be painless and the nodule or nodules will feel harder than other kinds of thyroid nodules. In addition, you may notice hard and swollen lymph glands near the thyroid resulting from the spread of the cancer within the neck. As is true for most forms of cancer, prompt recognition and treatment of thyroid cancer is important, for such tumors are usually curable. If your child has or is suspected of having a thyroid nodule, you should take the child to a physician for an examination. If the physician agrees that one or more nodules are present, he or she will perform studies necessary to determine the appropriate treatment, usually including thyroid blood tests and a thyroid scan. Often a thyroid biopsy can be performed in which a small piece of the nodule is obtained, usually enough to tell whether or not cancer is present. If cancer is found in a nodule, early treatment is imperative and should include an operation to remove as much malignant tissue as possible. Fortunately, this surgery is almost always successful and complete cure is likely. As with adults who have thyroid cancer, some children will also need treatment with radioactive iodine. In addition, lifelong treatment with thyroid hormone is always given to try to prevent further growth of any cancer cells that might remain. Your child will need periodic checkups after that, for thyroid cancer may reappear even in children taking thyroid hormone medication. If that happens, additional surgery or other treatments may be required.

If the nodule is benign, your physician will advise you if longterm treatment to *suppress* the thyroid is indicated. The pituitary gland normally stimulates and controls the thyroid by means of thyroid stimulating hormone. Since TSH tends to make nodules grow too, your physician may elect to treat your child with thyroid hormone tablets to shut off TSH production by the pituitary. Alternatively, your physician may prefer to see the child periodically and not treat with thyroid hormone unless the nodule enlarges or more nodules appear.

As we described in Chapter 10, there is a rare type of thyroid cancer known as *medullary carcinoma* that tends to run in families and that can be detected by means of a blood test for *calcitonin*, a hormone made by the tumor. People with this disease tend to have tumors of other glands as well, including the adrenal glands (which can cause high blood pressure), and parathyroid glands (which can raise the blood calcium level). Children who are found to have this type of cancer have their best chance for cure if it is discovered and removed early. Therefore, children in families in which this rare form of cancer has been found should have yearly calcitonin blood tests. When the tests suggest the presence of such a tumor, it should be removed at once.

In summary, if your child has a thyroid problem he or she may not look or act very sick. The only evidence that thyroid trouble is present may be a change in the child's growth rate. Therefore, the height and weight records that your pediatrician keeps often prove helpful in detecting thyroid disease. The treatments we use for thyroid disorders, including thyroid hormone, antithyroid drugs, radioactive iodine, and thyroid surgery, are effective and almost always curative. Unfortunately, each of these treatments has side effects that could be serious for some children. However, even though there is not one "best" treatment for your child's thyroid problem, it should be possible for you as a parent to understand why your child's physician recommends a particular way of treating that condition. The authors hope this chapter will help you to understand the recommendations made by your child's physician.

CHAPTER TWELVE

Childhood Head or Neck Irradiation

What May Happen Later

It must be appreciated that the usual course of growth of a thyroid cancer in young people is slow, and that the risk of death from thyroid cancer is extremely low. This risk must be balanced against the unavoidable risks which are associated with any medical intervention, including the development of undue anxiety, the cost and inconveniences of examinations, further radiation exposure, and the risk of surgery. Any medical procedures must be done after full and careful evaluation, recognizing that hasty action is very rarely required.

> Leslie J. DeGroot, M.D.
> Lawrence A. Frohman, M.D.
> Edwin L. Kaplan, M.D.
> Samuel Refetoff, M.D.

> —From the Summary of Conclusions of the Conference on Radiation-Associated Thyroid Cancer held at the University of Chicago in 1976

In the 1920s, physicians began to use radiation (x-rays) to treat noncancerous disorders.* One of the more common problems so treated was an enlargement of the thymus gland in the newborn. Other conditions treated in this manner included tonsils or adenoids, birthmarks, whooping cough, acne, and ringworm of the scalp.

*In this chapter we are referring to x-rays that were used to *treat* various medical problems. We are *not* referring to *diagnostic* x-rays, such as dental or chest x-rays.

Treatment was given earlier by means of an x-ray machine ("external beam irradiation") or by placing radioactive material, such as radium, directly in or on the tissue to be treated.

For many years, radiation was considered good medical therapy for some of these problems. For example, deafness was improved when radium treatments shrank enlarged lymph tissue compressing the internal ear canal. Acne could be markedly improved by radiation, resulting in less facial scarring. In short, radiation therapy was used because it seemed safe and effective.

Unfortunately, the thyroid gland, located as it is at the front of the neck, often received radiation inadvertently during treatment for these conditions. In the 1950s, physicians began to notice an increased number of benign and malignant thyroid tumors among patients who had been given radiation therapy years earlier. The fact that the radiation had caused the thyroid tumors was confirmed when it was found that many individuals exposed to atomic bomb radiation or fallout also developed thyroid tumors in later years. When these facts became known, these forms of radiation therapy were, of course, discontinued.* Nevertheless, it is estimated that between one and two million people across the United States received radiation treatments in childhood or adolescence between 1920 and 1960.

If you or a member of your family received such x-ray treatments in the past, it is possible that the hospital at which you were treated has tried to contact you to inform you about your radiation exposure. In fact, this effort on the part of hospitals has been remarkably effective, and many patients have already been contacted by mail. A typical letter from a hospital usually states the date and type of treatment, including the amount of radiation that was given. The letter probably

---

*Although radiation is no longer used to treat noncancerous conditions, it is now the mainstay of treatment for many forms of cancer.

recommends consultation with your family physician for an examination.

Unfortunately, since people tend to move many times during their lifetimes, and since women may change their names as well as their addresses, hospitals have been unable to reach many of these patients. Therefore, if you have not been contacted but think you have received x-ray treatment, please try to contact the hospital where your treatment was given. If the medical record of that treatment is still available, it will be forwarded to you promptly upon your request and will be helpful to the physician you go to for your follow-up examination. Here is an example of an appropriate letter to such a hospital:

Medical Record Department
Massachusetts General Hospital
Fruit Street
Boston, Massachusetts 02114

To the Medical Records Librarian:

I believe that I received x-ray treatment for an enlarged thymus gland a few days after I was born. Please send me my medical information about treatment given, including the dose of x-ray received, the number of treatments given, and the part of my body that was radiated.

My personal information is as follows:
Name at the time of treatment—Rebecca C. Smith
Date of Birth—March 21, 1926
Exact Date of Treatment—Unknown, probably late March 1926
Address at that time—27 Charles Street, Boston, MA
Mother's name—Mary Louise Smith
Father's name—Francis Clark Smith

Obstetrician—Grover Thornton, M.D.
Pediatrician—George Jones, M.D.

Very sincerely yours,
Rebecca Smith Jacobsen
323 Conant Road
Weston, MA 02193

It would be a good idea to enclose a stamped, self-addressed envelope, though under normal circumstances this would be provided by the hospital. In most cases, there will be no charge for this service.

Should you be unable to find the appropriate information in this manner, we would recommend that you make an effort to contact one of the physicians who treated you. Give the physician your name and address as it was at the time, since the information will be needed to locate your medical record. You may find that the doctor who treated you has died or moved away, or that your records have been lost or destroyed: but try to find them, for they can provide helpful information for the physician who will examine you.

If you had radiation treatments given to your head, neck, or chest, you may have many questions about their effect on you and what you should do about it. We are, in fact, still learning about the problem, so our answers should be considered provisional, reflecting our *present* state of knowledge in this area. As more information becomes known, our management of this common problem may, of course, change to some degree.

HOW COMMON IS THE APPEARANCE OF THYROID CANCER FOLLOWING EARLIER RADIATION?

If you had radiation treatment for an enlarged thymus, acne, or some other condition near your thyroid gland, you are more likely to develop thyroid cancer someday than someone who has no history of radiation treatment. Medical surveys suggest that your overall thyroid cancer risk is somewhere between 2 and 7 percent, compared with an annual incidence of 0.004 percent in the general population.[12] Furthermore, your risk increases with increased amounts of radiation. We have not observed an increased incidence of thyroid cancer in patients who had hyperthyroidism treated by radioactive iodine. Here the thyroid receives far greater amounts of radiation from the radioactive iodine treatment (from 4000 to 12,000 rads), and yet 30–40 years' follow-up of such patients has failed to demonstrate that they have an increased risk for thyroid cancer. However, recent reports suggest that high doses of *external* radiation, such as that given for certain forms of cancer, *can* cause thyroid tumors, as well as hypothyroidism.

WHAT OTHER FACTORS BESIDES THE AMOUNT OF RADIATION YOU RECEIVED INCREASE YOUR CHANCES OF DEVELOPING THYROID CANCER?

Clearly, one important factor is the *part of your body that was treated by x-rays*. Some patients received radiation by means of small pieces of radium placed directly in or on tissues to be treated. Radiation of tonsils or adenoid tissue was sometimes carried out in this manner. If that is your situation, your thyroid gland probably got less radiation effect than the thyroid of someone whose x-ray tratment was given directly to the front of the neck, where the thyroid is located.

We don't know whether your *age* at the time of radiation is a significant factor. Physicians originally thought that this might be the case, since experiments with animals generally indicate that the younger the animal is at the time of radiation, the more significant the effects of radiation may be. Therefore, we expected to find more thyroid tumors developing in patients who had radiation in infancy for thymic enlargement, than we did among patients who had radiation in teenage years for acne. Though our statistics are still incomplete, we can say at this time only that there is a significant amount of thyroid cancer in *both* groups of patients. On the other hand, there is some evidence that the younger an individual was at the time of radiation, the more likely that individual is to develop noncancerous (benign) thyroid nodules.[14] Finally, it is clear that the risk of developing thyroid problems stays with a person for his/her entire lifetime. Thyroid cancer has been detected in exposed individuals as long as 45 years after the x-ray treatments were administered.

A third factor currently under investigation is that of *hypothyroidism*. If a patient had radiation in childhood, and subsequently developed hypothyroidism (thyroid failure) as a second disorder, it is possible that the hypothyroidism itself may increase the risk of later development of thyroid nodules and thyroid cancer. This is because the pituitary gland secretes thyroid simulating hormone in response to the hypothyroidism. TSH is thought to be one factor that can cause thyroid tumors to develop. Experiments with animals suggest that is the case, although it has never been proved in human beings. Nevertheless, because of our experience with radiated animals, if even a slight decrease in thyroid function occurs in someone with a history of childhood radiation, it is very important to raise his or her thyroid blood level to normal through the administration of thyroid hormone tablets.

HAVE OTHER KINDS OF MEDICAL PROBLEMS APPEARED IN RADIATED PATIENTS?

Other kinds of neck tumors have been found in patients who received childhood radiation. These include tumors of the parotid (mumps) glands located in front of the ear, as well as the other salivary glands located beneath the jaw. In addition, tumors of the parathyroid glands, located behind the thyroid, appear to be found more commonly in radiated patients than in the general population. We are continuing to look for other associated medical problems, but as yet no other medical relationships have been firmly established.

WHAT SORT OF MEDICAL EXAMINATION IS ADVISED FOR PATIENTS WHO HAVE HAD CHILDHOOD RADIATION?

If you have had childhood radiation, you should be seen by your physician for yearly checkups. *Your physician will examine your neck* to determine whether thyroid nodules are present, and also to look for any abnormalities of your parotid glands, salivary glands, or lymph nodes that might suggest the presence of a tumor.

If a thyroid abnormality is found, a *thyroid scan* should be performed, both to evaluate the function of suspicious lumps and also to look for areas of diminished thyroid activity within your gland that could not be felt by your physician.

Because there is a lot that we don't know about the late effects of childhood radiation, readers will find a great deal of individual variation among physicians testing patients with a history of childhood radiation. For example, at the Massachusetts General Hospital it is our practice to carry out a thyroid scan on *all* patients with a history of childhood irradiation when they are first seen. We do this even if we cannot feel any nodules because we want to know if there are areas of diminished function within the thyroid that we should be especially careful to observe for the later development of thyroid tumors. A thyroid scan, using techniques currently available, adds very little radiation to your already-radiated thyroid gland. As explained in reference note 2, in the Reference and Comment section of the book, the thyroid receives a dose of 0.5 to 2.0 rads from radioiodine (^{123}I) and 0.2 to 1.8 rads from radioactive technetium (^{99m}Tc). Your physician may not perform such a scan on you, however, if your thyroid feels normal and you are willing to return for periodic examinations.

Your physician will probably perform a blood test to measure your level of thyroid hormone (T_4) as well as your level of pituitary thyroid stimulating hormone (TSH) to look for evidence of hypothyroidism. We do this because hypothyroidism clearly increases the risk of thyroid cancer in radiated animals. Although that risk has not been proved in human beings, we do not want to take any chances. Your physician may recommend further tests depending on the findings of your particular examination.

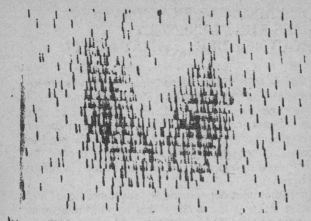

Figure 30   A normal thyroid scan.

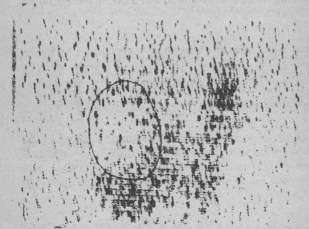

Figure 31   A thyroid scan showing a nonfunctioning or "cold" nodule.

IF YOUR MEDICAL EXAMINATION REVEALS THE PRESENCE OF A THYROID NODULE ... WHAT NEXT?

If your doctor feels a thyroid nodule and it shows diminished function on thyroid scan (Figures 30 and 31), it should be either biopsied* or entirely removed to be sure that it is not cancerous. In contrast, nodules that appear to function normally on scan do not necessarily need to be removed, although they should be followed carefully and reexamined in one year (or sooner, at the discretion of the physician).

Further treatment depends on the results of the T_4 and TSH blood tests. If these show that hypothyroidism is present,* treatment will be with thyroid hormone tablets in increasing doses until the serum TSH becomes undetectable (see Chapter 6).[15]

WHAT SORT OF CONTINUED HEALTH CHECKUPS SHOULD YOU HAVE IF YOU WERE TREATED WITH RADIATION IN CHILDHOOD?

The nature of your follow-up evaluation depends on what was found at the time of your initial evaluation. If your initial examination reveals *no thyroid nodule*, and your thyroid blood tests and scan are normal, you can

---

*By *biopsy* we are referring to either of two related procedures: "needle biopsy" (done with a large hollow needle by means of which a core of tissue is obtained) and "fine needle aspiration" (done with a small needle by means of which thyroid cells are obtained). (See Chapter 10 for a full description of thyroid biopsies.)

*Hypothyroidism is more likely if you received radiation as part of cancer treatment rather than for a noncancerous condition.

simply have yearly checkups by your family physician, with thyroid blood tests to be sure that you do not develop hypothyroidism. It is *not* recommended that a thyroid scan be done every year, since the scan itself radiates the thyroid to a small extent.

On the other hand, if your initial thyroid evaluation revealed the presence of *one or more small nodules*, a different follow-up is usually indicated. If there is no evidence that the nodule(s) are functioning excessively, your physician will probably attempt to *suppress* their growth with thyroid hormone tablets. As explained in Chapter 10, such treatment with thyroid tablets raises your blood level of thyroid hormone, which blocks the release of thyroid stimulating hormone from your pituitary. TSH tends to make many thyroid nodules grow larger, and shutting off TSH often makes thyroid nodules shrink. If there is no diminution in size after three to six months of such treatment, however, your physician will probably recommend that the nodule(s) be removed surgically.

It should be stressed that your risk of developing thyroid tumors following childhood radiation does *not* disappear with time. Therefore you must continue to have yearly checkups of your thyroid gland *throughout your lifetime*. Needless to say, we expect to improve our treatment and follow-up programs as we learn more about radiation-related thyroid disease.

CONTROVERSIAL "CANCERS"

In our discussion about thyroid tumors and cancers, we have been referring, in general, to nodules that are larger than 1.5 centimeters (½ inch) in diameter. One of the most hotly contested issues in the field of thyroid cancer has to do with the presence in many thyroid glands of very small tumors that are smaller than 1.5 centimeters in size, some so small that they can be detected only with a microscope. And though many of these abnormal areas look like cancers, there is no proof that they actually ever develop into a growing, spreading cancer. Since they can occur in individuals who have never had childhood radiation, as well as in those who were exposed to x-ray treatments in childhood, we see no reason to recommend removal of a thyroid gland simply because of the possible presence of such areas and a history of childhood radiation.

Much work is continuing at medical centers all over the world to understand this and the other controversial areas mentioned within this chapter. Frankly, the fact that so many controversies still exist is a very good reason for a periodic checkup with your doctor if you have had childhood irradiation. Every effort is being made by groups like the American Thyroid Association and the American Cancer Society to keep you and your physician well-informed as the state of our knowledge improves.

CHAPTER THIRTEEN

Thyroid Trouble in Pregnancy

If you are pregnant, the changes that are happening in your body because of the pregnancy may make it difficult for both you and your physician to tell if something is happening to your thyroid too. For example, an overactive thyroid may make you feel nervous, overheated, shaky, and flushed, all of which may happen to a woman in normal pregnancy who has a healthy thyroid. Furthermore, since your physician must consider the baby inside you, the thyroid tests and treatment for you will be different from what they would be if you were not pregnant. Despite these difficulties, if you do develop a problem with your thyroid gland during pregnancy, it can be diagnosed correctly and treated successfully.

Increased amounts of female sex hormones circulate in your blood during pregnancy, causing your blood level of thyroid hormone to rise. However, although the *total* amount of thyroid hormone is increased, the extra thyroid hormone is in an inactive condition *bound* to certain proteins in your blood and therefore has no effect on you or your unborn child. If we measure the concentration of active or *unbound* thyroid hormone in the blood of a healthy pregnant woman, it proves to be no different from the level in a healthy nonpregnant woman.

It used to be common for the thyroid to enlarge during pregnancy. However, current medical evidence indicates that the size of your thyroid probably does not change much in pregnancy if you live in one of the developed areas of the world where diets contain plenty of iodine. In the United States, for example, iodine deficiency does not occur in pregnancy, because our diets contain adequate amounts of iodine, and in addition, most vitamins prescribed during pregnancy also contain iodine. Therefore, if you live in this country and develop a goiter in pregnancy, it is likely that you have a thyroid problem. In that case, your obstetrician probably will arrange for you to have thyroid tests performed. Alternatively, you may be referred to a specialist for your thyroid evaluation.

THE OVERACTIVE THYROID IN PREGNANCY

Hyperthyroidism is not a particularly common condition among pregnant women, since hyperthyroid women often do not have normal reproductive cycles and therefore have difficulty both in becoming pregnant and in maintaining a normal pregnancy. However, if you do have an overactive thyroid, and if your thyroid remains markedly overactive throughout your pregnancy, your baby is a little more likely to be premature and small than if your thyroid were normal. On the other hand, if your thyroid is only slightly overactive, or if it can be controlled during pregnancy, there is no added risk to you and little, if any, danger to your baby.

Hyperthyroidism can be difficult to recognize in pregnancy, since many of the symptoms and signs of hyperthyroidism occur in normal pregnancy. Pregnant women may normally experience a fast pulse, nervousness, heat intolerance, flushing, and increased perspiration. Hyperthyroidism, therefore, may seem like no more than an exaggeration of these "normal" signs of a healthy pregnancy. Usually, however, there are other clues that the thyroid is overactive. Your heart rate may be especially fast—more than 120 beats per minute. You may fail to gain weight, and may even lose weight as calories are burned up at a rapid rate. Finally, your thyroid may enlarge as it becomes overactive.

If your obstetrician suspects that you have hyperthyroidism, it is usually easy to diagnose by means of blood tests that measure the level of your thyroid hormone. If your thyroid is overactive, the level should be higher than the modest elevation seen in normal pregnancy. Moreover, the active (unbound) thyroid hormone level usually will be significantly elevated above normal. Radioactive iodine cannot be used as a further test for hyperthyroidism if you are pregnant, because it would be passed from your body across the placenta to your baby and might damage its thyroid tissue. If the diagnosis is in doubt, your obstetrician may simply wait and repeat thyroid blood tests a few weeks later, since a mild degree of hyperthyroidism docs not appear to pose a significant danger to either you or your unborn child.[16]

Two antithyroid drugs may be used to treat hyperthyroidism: propylthiouracil (PTU) and methimazole (Tapazole), both of which block the manufacture of thyroid hormone by the thyroid gland. Since these drugs can cross from your system into your baby's blood stream and affect your baby's thyroid gland, your treatment dosage must be kept to a minimum. At first, enough of the drug must be given to bring your hyperthyroidism under control. As soon as that control has been achieved, however, the dosage is reduced to the lowest possible amount that will keep you healthy and yet minimize the drug effect on your unborn child. In practice, this usually means a total daily dose of less than 200 milligrams of propylthiouracil or 20 milligrams of methimazole,* though sometimes it is possible to reduce the amount of antithyroid drug even further in the later

---

*The authors use propylthiouracil exclusively in pregnancy because of several reports that suggest that minor birth defects occasionally may occur with methimazole treatment.

stages of pregnancy, when hyperthyroidism often seems to become milder.

Some patients taking propylthiouracil or methimazole may become allergic to these drugs and develop a red skin rash, itching, or hives. More rarely, these drugs can cause a dangerous decrease in certain white blood cells (neutrophils) that normally help control infections. Therefore, if you are taking one of these drugs and develop a rash, itching, hives, or evidence of an infection (such as a fever or sore throat), you should *immediately* stop the drug and contact your physician *that day*. If you have a fever or sore throat you will need to have a blood test to be sure that an infection has not developed due to a lowering of your white cell count. If the neutrophil count is normal and there is no evidence of drug allergy, your physician will probably restart your antithyroid drug even while you are being treated for the infection. If, on the other hand, your neutrophil count is low, or your physician finds other evidence of drug allergy, another form of treatment for your hyperthyroidism must be chosen.

Propranolol (Inderal), which blocks the action of the thyroid hormone on the body, may be used in pregnancy for short periods of time to help control symptoms of hyperthyroidism. This drug is extremely successful in slowing a fast pulse rate and reducing nervousness and anxiety, but it has unfortunate side effects that keep us from using it for a long period of time during pregnancy. Propranolol may slow the growth and development of your unborn baby. Furthermore, some medical reports suggest that if you are taking propranolol at the end of pregnancy your baby may be born with difficulty in breathing, a slow pulse, a low blood sugar. For these reasons, we prefer to use propranolol only briefly and early in pregnancy and only if the hyperthyroidism is severe.

In some instances, a physician will recommend an operation to remove your thyroid gland as a way of treating hyperthyroidism when you are pregnant. If so, the surgery usually will be delayed until after the third month of pregnancy, because any kind of surgery earlier in pregnancy is associated with a slightly increased risk of miscarriage. A few weeks' treatment with an antithyroid drug or a few days' treatment with the thyroid hormone blocking drug propranolol are usually given to control the overactive thyroid before your thyroid operation is performed. Iodine, which might ordinarily be prescribed, is not used to prepare a pregnant woman for thyroid surgery, since it would affect the baby's thyroid, too. In like manner, *radioactive* iodine cannot be used to treat hyperthyroidism during pregnancy, for the radioiodine would cross from you into your baby and damage the baby's thyroid.

If you have been hyperthyroid during your pregnancy (or at any time earlier in your life) your doctor will examine your baby for hyperthyroidism. This condition may occur when the thyroid stimulators that cause your own thyroid to be overactive cross the placenta to your unborn baby in large enough quantities to stimulate your baby's thyroid to overactivity too. Fortunately this condition is extremely rare and develops in only about one in every 70 babies born to hyperthyroid mothers.[17] If such a condition is found it is usually mild, requires no treatment, and subsides in a few weeks. If it is severe, however, it may cause thyroid enlargement and make the infant sick with marked irritability and a very rapid heartbeat, and may interfere with the baby's growth in the first days and weeks of life. If so, the baby's thyroid overactivity can be controlled with medication until it subsides (see Chapter 11).

If you took antithyroid drugs during pregnancy, the doctors will also examine your baby for evidence of an underactive thyroid (hypothyroidism) and thyroid enlargement (goiter). If either condition has been caused by your medications, treatment is not usually required, since the problem will disappear rapidly as these drugs leave your baby's body.

On the other hand, one in every 4000 to 5000 babies is

born with hypothyroidism due to an underlying thyroid problem of its own. That kind of hypothyroidism will *not* go away by itself and therefore must be recognized and treated as early as possible. Fortunately thyroid tests are now performed on most newborn babies in this country so that they are more apt to be found and successfully treated before permanent harm is done.[18]

If you have been hyperthyroid during a pregnancy, your thyroid condition should be carefully watched in the weeks following the birth of your baby. Your thyroid may gradually become more overactive following delivery. If so, and if you are breast-feeding your baby, your physician must still consider your baby's welfare in deciding how to continue to treat your thyroid. It is generally advised that if you are breast-feeding you should not take the antithyroid drugs propylthiouracil or methimazole, since both appear in breast milk. Once ingested by the baby, it is possible they will interfere with your infant's thyroid gland. However, the amounts of these drugs that get into breast milk are very small, and probably pose little risk to the child. So if you strongly desire to nurse while taking these drugs you may do so, but close monitoring of your infant's thyroid hormone levels and white blood cell count is essential.

It is of great importance that you not be treated for hyperthyroidism with radioactive iodine while you are breast-feeding, for in such a case some of the radioactive iodine would be passed on to your baby in your milk. The amount of radioactive iodine that your baby would receive in this manner might cause subsequent harm to its thyroid.[19] Therefore, if you are breast-feeding and *must* be given radioactive iodine to control an overactive thyroid you will find that your physician will ask you to stop breast-feeding before the treatment is given and until the radioactivity has disappeared from your milk.

THE UNDERACTIVE THYROID IN PREGNANCY

If your physician suspects that you may have an underactive thyroid, he or she will measure your blood level of thyroid stimulating hormone as well as your blood level of thyroid hormone. Since the elevated levels of sex hormones that occur in pregnancy cause the thyroid hormone level to rise, it is possible for a pregnant woman with an *underactive* thyroid to have what seems to be a normal blood level of thyroid hormone, which could cause an error or delay in the discovery of a thyroid deficiency. But although the total thyroid hormone level is normal, the "free" or "unbound" level is below normal. (See Chapter 2 for a more complete discussion of this point.) Fortunately, an elevation of TSH is a highly reliable indication of an underactive thyroid. TSH is the pituitary gland hormone that normally controls your thyroid gland. If your thyroid gland fails, and your free thyroid hormone level falls below normal, your pituitary will make more TSH. In such a case your blood level of TSH will be increased even if pregnancy keeps your total blood level of thyroid hormone in the "normal range."

If you are found to have hypothyroidism while you are pregnant there is no need for alarm, though of course the condition should be treated when the diagnosis is made. Your baby has its own thyroid and should be fine.[19] Furthermore your condition should improve rapidly as soon as your physician treats you with thyroid hormone tablets to bring your hormone to a level that is appropriate for pregnancy. Then your TSH will be checked to be certain that you are taking enough thyroid medication. The TSH level will be normal if your treatment is adequate.

THYROID NODULES IN PREGNANCY

Thyroid lumps or nodules in pregnancy present a special problem because radioactive iodine scans cannot be used as a way of evaluating their function. The radioactive iodine used in such scanning procedures would be a risk to your unborn child, whose thyroid might be damaged even by a low dose of radioiodine. Actually, the baby's thyroid doesn't take up iodine until about the tenth week of pregnancy, but any radiation exposure to the fetus should be avoided if possible.

If you do develop a thyroid nodule during pregnancy, other tests can be done that will tell why the nodule has developed, and yet will not endanger you or your child. Thyroid blood tests can indicate whether your nodule is associated with a more general condition, such as an overactive or underactive thyroid. A thyroid ultrasound test can be used to tell whether a nodule is solid or is a fluid-filled cyst. Most important, a thyroid needle biopsy usually can be performed with complete safety during the pregnancy, and an examination of the tissue obtained should reveal the cause of the nodule.

If a biopsy shows that your thyroid nodule is harmless, it can be left alone or treated with thyroid hormone. If the nodule is found to contain cancer, it can be removed in an operation, preferably after the third month of the pregnancy, when there is the least risk to your baby from any surgical procedure. In addition, thyroid hormone treatment can be given to help control the cancer, just as in a nonpregnant patient with such a tumor.

In summary, if you have a thyroid problem during pregnancy, it can be diagnosed and treated effectively even though the hormonal changes that occur in pregnancy may alter your thyroid blood tests to some degree. The treatment of your thyroid condition in pregnancy is similar to that given to nonpregnant women, though in some situations treatment may be modified to avoid endangering your unborn child. When the baby is born, he or she will be carefully examined for evidence of a thyroid problem and will almost certainly have a thyroid blood test performed as a routine measure.

TABLE 4

The Effect of Alteration in Dietary Iodine Intake

Recommended Range of Daily Iodine Intake:
150–300 micrograms*/day
Actual Range of Daily Iodine Intake—U.S.A.:
200–700 micrograms/day

ILLNESS CAUSED BY ALTERED IODINE INTAKE

TOO LITTLE IODINE

Less than 25 micrograms Iodine/day	Some children born with goiter, hypothyroidism, retardation, cretinism.
Less than 50 micrograms Iodine/day	Goiter in some adults.

TOO MUCH IODINE

Approximately 1 milligram daily	May cause *hyperthyroidism* in elderly people who have nodular goiters.
Approximately 10 milligrams daily	Some babies born with *goiter* if mother takes this much iodine during pregnancy.
Approximately 20 milligrams daily	Some people with Graves' disease can become *hypothyroid*—more likely if they have had radioiodine treatment or surgical removal of part of their thryoid in the past.

Approximately 200 milligrams daily

Healthy people: slight change in thyroid hormone level but still feel well.

Newborn babies: may be *hypothyroid* at birth.

People with Hashimoto's disease (chronic thyroiditis): 50 percent become *hypothyroid*.

Patient with Graves' disease (diffuse toxic goiter): *hypothyroidism* common, especially in those previously treated with radioiodine or a thyroid operation.

Patients with nodular goiter: 50 percent become *hyperthyroid* (some do so on much less iodine—see above).

*1000 micrograms = 1 milligram
  1000 milligrams = 1 gram
     28.4 grams = 1 ounce

  **One kelp tablet usually contains 150 micrograms of iodine.

  5 drops of "Saturated Solution of Potassium Iodide" (given as an expectorant) contain 180 milligrams of iodine.

  A kidney x-ray (IVP) gives you 10–20 grams of iodine.

  A gall bladder x-ray (cholecystogram) gives about 2 grams of iodine.

  Other iodine-containing medications include Quadrinal, Ornade, and Organidin used for coughs and colds, Combid given for stomach problems, and Amiodarone, which is prescribed for some heart patients. Many vitamin-mineral preparations also contain 150–300 micrograms of iodine per capsule —a potential danger for those who take them in large amounts.

CHAPTER FOURTEEN

Effect of Drugs, Food, Stress, and Radiation on the Thyroid

A person develops exophthalmic goiter after a fright because he is a special type of person. Another might develop asthma or peptic ulcer or manic depressive psychosis after an identical experience. Many more would develop nothing more than very temporary "jitters." We must look upon the development of exophthalmic goiter after psychic trauma as the result of a stimulus applied to an individual preconditioned to make that remarkable response. The patient is a loaded gun. The psychic trauma pulls the trigger.

—J. H. Means, *The Thyroid and Its Diseases* (New York: J. B. Lippincott Co., 1937), page 565.

DRUGS

Iodine

Iodine is the cause of more thyroid problems than all other food substances combined. You can get sick from eating either too much or too little iodine. In a few countries, especially in remote mountainous areas where the daily iodine intake is less than 25 micrograms per day, the lack of enough iodine commonly causes thyroid enlargement (goiter) in addition to mental and physical retardation among the population.

In contrast, in the United States you eat more iodine than is really necessary. The Food and Nutrition Board of the National Research Council has recommended a daily intake of 150 to 300 micrograms of iodine per day, but if you live in the United States your daily dietary iodine intake is probably between 200 and 700 micrograms per day. This is because extra iodine has been added to bread, milk, salt, and other foods that you consume frequently. Normal individuals seem to have the ability to control the amount of iodine that actually enters their thyroid gland even if their diet is supplemented with extra iodine. However, as shown in Table 4, if you have a problem with your thyroid, that problem could make you more likely to develop a change in thyroid function if you take in too much iodine in your diet or in other ways. That would be true, for example, if you ever had hyperthyroidism due to a generalized overactivity of your thyroid gland (diffuse toxic goiter or Graves' disease) or if you have a low-grade inflammation of your thyroid known as chronic lymphocytic thyroiditis (Hashimoto's disease). Either condition would give you a tendency to develop *hypo*thyroidism if you were exposed to even a modest amount of extra iodine. In fact, patients who have had Graves' disease have become hypothyroid after ingesting as little as 18 milligrams of iodine per day.

Unborn babies are also very sensitive to iodine excess. Therefore, if you are pregnant and ingest large quantities of iodine in the form of a medication or kelp (seaweed), you risk having your baby born with a goiter and possibly with an underactive thyroid as well. A large goiter could compress the baby's windpipe and interfere with breathing. Moreover, since iodine can also be transmitted from mother to child in breast milk, you should avoid health foods and medications that contain extra iodine while nursing your baby.

An *abrupt* increase in dietary iodine can cause *hyper*thyroidism in people living in iodine-deficient areas of the world. "Epidemics" of hyperthyroidism have been seen in several countries when iodine was added to the national diet to correct a long-standing problem of widespread iodine deficiency. This happened in the U.S. in the 1920s when health authorities added iodine to salt.

Hyperthyroidism caused by excess iodine also has been observed in the United States and other parts of the world where dietary iodine is sufficient. In such areas, older patients with lumpy thyroids (nodular goiters) are those most likely to be affected by an increase in iodine intake. Moreover, since these patients tend to be elderly, they are more likely to have complications from the rapid pulse or irregular heart rhythm that may happen when their thyroid becomes overactive.

Therefore, if you have Graves' or Hashimoto's disease, are pregnant or nursing a baby, or if you have a nodular goiter, you should try to avoid an abrupt increase in your iodine intake. Do *not* eat kelp, and do read labels on bottles of vitamins and other medications. If you are having an x-ray for which a dye is given to you by mouth or by injection, find out if there is iodine in the x-ray dye. This is likely if the x-ray is of your kidney, spinal canal, gall bladder, or blood vessels. This is not to say you cannot take a medication that contains iodine or that you shouldn't have one of these special x-rays. Rather, if that is your situation, your doctor may choose to examine you after you take the medication or have the x-ray to be sure that your thyroid function has not changed.

The natural iodine of most foods is low. It is highest in seafoods, and there are variable amounts of bread, milk, eggs, and meat. Fruits contain little iodine, as do vegetables with the exception of spinach. The exact amounts of iodine in these foodstuffs vary so widely and depend on so many factors that it is no longer possible to make a satisfactory list of the iodine content of foods.[21] Instead, the message here is to eat a "regular diet" during pregnancy and while breast-feeding or if you know you have a thyroid condition. You do not need to avoid iodized salt, bread, and seafood—just don't take in *extra* iodine if possible in medications or special foods like kelp. But if such foods or medications must be taken, they can be used under your doctor's supervision.*

If you or your physician wants to know more about iodine intake the best thing to do is to measure the iodine content of your urine. In a general way the amount of iodine in your urine is equal to the amount you take in from all sources, including food, medications, and special x-ray dyes. Such a test could be helpful if you are pregnant and want to know exactly how much iodine you are taking in. However, in most cases that information is far less important than a measurement of your thyroid hormone and TSH blood levels.

Lithium

Lithium is a drug that is being used increasingly (and quite effectively) to treat certain types of mental illness. Lithium has been shown to affect thyroid gland function and size in some patients. The same patients who get goiter and hypothyroidism from iodine—those with a history of hyperthyroidism due to Graves' disease and thyroiditis due to Hashimoto's disease—are also the most likely to have these problems from lithium. However, even if you have Graves' or Hashimoto's disease, you can still take lithium safely. If you need to take lithium, your physician will probably examine your thyroid and check your thyroid hormone (T_4) and TSH level after you have been taking lithium for a few weeks. If thyroid deficiency is found, you do not need to stop lithium, for supplemental thyroid hormone administration can correct your deficiency and permit you to continue to take this useful drug.

---

*For example, the drug amiodarone used to treat irregular heart rhythms contains enough iodine to affect thyroid function in some patients. You can take amiodarone if needed, however, as long as you doctor checks your blood level of thyroid hormone and prescribes medication to correct thyroid abnormalities if they occur.

FOOD

Much has been written about the effect of food upon the thyroid yet most of what you eat does not present a danger to you. Kelp may contain large amounts of iodine, which is discussed in the preceding section. Foods of the Brassica family (including cabbage, kale, rutabaga, turnips) contain a substance that is capable of causing goiter in both animals and humans. Medical research suggests that these foods cause goiter and a decrease in thyroid function because they produce a chemical compound known as *goitrin*, which we know has a negative effect on the thyroid. However, even though these foods may produce goiter in people who live in iodine-deficient areas, we are not aware of anyone in whom the thyroid has actually become underactive just because these foods were eaten.

Some years ago, infants who were allergic to milk were given formulas prepared with soy protein instead of milk. Some of these babies developed goiter and thyroid deficiency. The problem was corrected when extra iodine was added to the soy formulas. Soy formulas are still in use and, with the added iodine, no longer cause thyroid problems in the babies who take them.

STRESS

Physicians have long suspected that stress might play a role in causing the type of hyperthyroidism in which the whole thyroid becomes overactive (diffuse toxic goiter or Graves' disease). Distressing experiences, usually involving a personal loss (such as the death of a loved one or a divorce), often precede the onset of hyperthroidism and may act as "trigger factors" that precipitate thyroid overactivity in genetically susceptible individuals.

Investigators have found other evidence of a relationship between stress and the thyroid. For example, an increase in hyperthyroidism occurred among refugees from Nazi prison camps, as well as among the inhabitants of occupied Denmark during World War II. There have also been experimental studies that have shown changes in thyroid function in animals subjected to stressful conditions. In spite of all our efforts, however, we still do not know *how* such stress affects the thyroid —just that it seems to "trigger off" thyroid overactivity in some susceptible people.

Physical stresses—such as serious infection, pregnancy, or a surgical operation—may also play a role in the onset of hyperthyroidism in certain individuals. Here, too, although some thyroid specialists accept the idea that such a relationship may exist, we do not know how these physical happenings exert their effect on thyroid function.

ENVIRONMENTAL FACTORS

Much investigation has been carried out to try to understand the effects of such factors as cold, heat, and exercise on the function of your thyroid. This research has shown that none of these environmental factors appears to influence thyroid function to a degree that would significantly affect you even if you had an underlying thyroid problem. Thus, your requirement for thyroid hormone does not change in response to a hotter or colder climate, a change in temperature or altitude, or a change in your physical activity.

RADIATION*

Benign and malignant thyroid disease following exposure of the thyroid to external radiation in childhood has been

*For a more detailed and comprehensive discussion of the risks of radiation, please refer to Chapter 12.

the subject of an entire chapter in this book. A similar pattern of disease can occur if your thyroid is exposed to radiation at any age, and this subject is therefore of vital concern to physicians. This is particularly true now that nuclear medicine and radiation therapy are playing important roles in the diagnosis and treatment of many diseases.

Your thyroid can be exposed to radiation in two ways. When x-ray treatments are given externally to your neck area, your thyroid may be exposed if it is in the pathway of the radiation. This form of radiation can cause thyroid tumors many years after exposure. A second sort of radiation exposure occurs when your thyroid takes up radioactive iodine and is thus exposed from *within*. Since your thyroid uses iodine in the manufacture of thyroid hormones, any radioactive iodine that gets into your body will go to your thyroid gland by way of your blood stream. Then, from within the gland, the atoms of radioactive iodine can produce local radiation effects on nearby thyroid cells. This process continues until iodine is discharged from your gland or loses its radioactivity by *decay*.

Small doses of this "internal" thyroid radiation are not necessarily harmful, and are definitely *less* harmful than comparable doses of external radiation. Radioiodine forms the basis of several thyroid tests as well as treatment of hyperthyroidism and thyroid cancer. In these situations, physicians administer radioactive iodine either to visualize your thyroid or to damage overactive or cancerous thyroid tissues. Because only the thyroid takes up iodine, the rest of the body is largely spared from unnecessary exposure to radiation.

On the other hand, it is possible that a nuclear reactor accident could release *large* amounts of radioactive iodine into the atmosphere. If you were to inhale that radioiodine, it could get into your system and accumulate in your thyroid gland. The radioactive iodine might then damage your thyroid tissue or lead to the formation of benign or cancerous thyroid tumors. The nature of the radiation effects would depend upon how much radio-iodine reached your thyroid and how long it remained there.

Fortunately, nonradioactive potassium iodide can be taken by mouth to dilute the effects of the radioactive iodine, but in order for it to be effective, it must be taken within the first three to four hours after exposure to the radioactive iodine and must be continued daily for the next three to ten days.

The Bureau of Radiation Health and the Bureau of Drugs of the U.S. Food and Drug Administration are currently preparing detailed guidelines for the administration of potassium iodide in the event of a nuclear emergency. Clearly, people living near a nuclear reactor should have the potassium iodide readily available in their homes to be taken promptly upon notification of an accident that has released dangerous amounts* of radio-iodine into the atmosphere. The recommended daily dosage of potassium iodide for children under one year of age is likely to be 65 milligrams, and 130 milligrams for everyone else. This amount of iodine, easily taken by mouth once a day, is adequate to keep the radioactive iodine out of the thyroid and yet is not enough to cause trouble for people who might be sensitive to iodine (infants, pregnant women, and elderly people with nodular thyroid glands—as described earlier in this chapter).

These general concepts of radiation safety are sure to be clarified in detail by forthcoming government documents and recommendations by local health authorities in areas where nuclear reactors are located.

OTHER CONSIDERATIONS

A variety of other drugs and environmental factors have been shown to affect the thyroid in some individuals or

---

*Enough radioiodine to expose thyroid glands of humans to at least 10 to 20 rads of radiation.

to change the thyroid function of animals in experimental situations. Fortunately, the medical community is very much aware that any new drug must be carefully tested for possible adverse effects of any kind on the body. Indeed, such tests, following the guidelines of the Food and Drug Administration, are proving generally effective in preventing thyroid problems in patients taking new drugs. Where problems exist, a treatment is usually available, as is the case when goiter or hypothyroidism develop in patients taking lithium. As a general precaution, however, when you have your periodic health examination, you should be sure to tell your physician about all the drugs, vitamins, and health foods you are taking.

CHAPTER FIFTEEN

Is Your Thyroid Making You Fat?

This chapter is written for you if you are overweight and were told in the past that you were fat because you had an underactive thyroid. Our purpose here is twofold: first, to help you understand why you were told you were hypothyroid in the first place, and second, to help you find out whether you really are hypothyroid now.

When you develop hypothyroidism, you do *not*, as a rule, also become fat. Your body's use of oxygen (its metabolic rate) decreases, and you may become less physically active than you were when your thyroid was normal; but you probably will not eat enough food to gain a lot of weight. Furthermore, when you are started on thyroid hormone treatment for hypothyroidism, you are not likely to lose much weight, even if you were markedly obese to begin with. There may be a weight loss of three to four pounds early in treatment, but that is due to a loss of accumulated tissue fluid, rather than a loss of fat.

Nevertheless, you may be taking thyroid hormone tablets today because you, like many other people, were told in the past that you had an underactive thyroid that was causing obesity. Perhaps you will recall having a "breathing test" (Basal Metabolic Rate test or BMR) or a blood test for protein-bound iodine (PBI), which was interpreted by your physician as being low or in a "borderline range." If you lost weight in the weeks after thyroid hormone treatment was begun, you were probably told that your "clinical trial" on thyroid hormone treatment confirmed the fact that you were indeed hypothyroid.

However, the BMR and PBI tests were not sensitive enough to make a definite diagnosis of hypothyroidism, especially if your thyroid function was only slightly diminished. Obesity itself lowers the BMR and may have given a false impression of hypothyroidism. Physicians now rely on a low blood level of thyroid hormone (thyroxine or T_4) and an elevated blood level of the pituitary's thyroid stimulating hormone to make the diagnosis of mild hypothryoidism. The TSH level, by far the most sensitive indicator of thyroid failure, rises when your pituitary releases TSH into the blood stream because it senses that there is too little thyroid hormone in your blood. Before 1970 it was not possible to measure your serum TSH. Your physician had to rely on less sensitive tests, clinical judgment, and your response to thyroid hormone treatment. Of course, at the time you were first tested, you may have been hypothyroid, and you may still have that problem today. On the other hand, you may have always had a normal thyroid gland.

If you lost weight taking thyroid hormone medication, it may have been due to a carefully kept diet rather than to any effect of your thyroid treatment. You also may have experienced a *placebo* effect from your thyroid tablets: *Believing* the tablets would help you lose weight helped you achieve weight loss.

By measuring your serum TSH level now, it is possible to tell with certainty whether you are hypothyroid. This is important to do for three reasons. *First*, if the diagnosis of hypothyroidism was made by older, less sensitive tests, it is worthwhile to find out if there really is a thyroid problem, for if your thyroid is normal, there is no need to spend money on thyroid medication. Even if you have taken thyroid medication for many years, you can stop it and normal thyroid function will return rapidly if you do not really need it. *Second*, an excessive dose of thyroid hormone can be a health hazard to you if you are elderly, causing such symptoms as irregular or rapid heartbeat, muscle weakness, nervousness, and difficulty sleeping. *Third*, if you do have hypothyroidism, you should continue to take thyroid hormone pills for the rest of your life. Your thyroid hormone and TSH blood levels should be measured periodically by your family physician to be sure that your dosage of thyroid hormone is correct. This is important because patients who are mildly hypothyroid when young often experience a greater degree of thyroid deficiency in later life, and require a gradual increase in their dosage of thyroid hormone. For these reasons, if you were given thyroid hormone many years ago as treatment for an underactive thyroid or obesity, you should find out now whether your thyroid is normal or not. If it is normal, medication is unnecessary. If it is not normal, your physician can test you and determine what your proper dose of thyroid hormone should be.

Your physician can easily and safely find out whether you need thyroid treatment by asking you to stop taking your thyroid medication. Six weeks later, a sample of your blood can be tested for T_4 and TSH. The T_4 serves as a general indicator of your thyroid function. It should be low if you are very hypothyroid, but it may be within the "normal range" if your thyroid is only mildly underactive. Your TSH, on the other hand, will *always* be increased above normal if you are hypothyroid, even in a mild degree. Furthermore, your serum TSH can be used as a guide to find the correct dose of thyroid hormone for you. Your TSH will be normal if your thyroid is healthy, even if you have taken thyroid hormone tablets for many years.

In summary, if you are a patient who is taking thyroid hormone in the belief that it helps you deal with a weight problem, you are probably wrong. Rather, if you are controlling your weight, the credit is due to you, not the thyroid pills. Nevertheless, it is important to find out whether or not your thyroid is normal. By stopping the thyroid treatment, a blood test for thyroxine and TSH, drawn under supervision of your physician, will show you whether or not you need such medication. If you need thyroid hormone, the dosage should be correctly given and periodically rechecked. If you don't need it, thyroid tablets represent an unnecessary expense and potential health hazard.

OBESITY*

by T. D.

I am presently on my longest and most successful diet to date. However, I've been dieting, with varying degrees of success, for at least ten years. I've fasted, taken diet pills and tranquilizers, drunk ten glasses of water a day, joined Weight Watchers, and eaten grapefruit each meal. I've joined a diet workshop, done the Canadian Air Force Exercises, eaten Ayds (I ate a whole box in two days; they tasted great since I wasn't eating much food), joined Weight Watchers again, cut out breakfast, cut out lunch, cut out snacks. I've been offered a new summer wardrobe, a winter, spring, and fall wardrobe. I guess if there were any justice in this world, and starting a diet counted for, say, minus five pounds, I'd weigh a hundred pounds today. But I don't (yet). Starting a diet obviously doesn't count. Staying on one does. It's that simple, but it's hard.

Why do I start a diet? I haven't had any of those dramatic, impressive, catastrophic reasons that we've all heard of. I've never been unable to buckle an airline seatbelt, or had a heart attack, or been caught in a revolving door, or been unable to find anything to fit me while shopping. There's always Lane Bryant's Chubby Shop. For me, it's usually been an accumulation of things: Never looking as good or as well tailored as my roommate. (Why do fat people always have thin roommates?) Standing pretty much alone at a college mixer,

*We include this creative comment about obesity for our readers' interest, since most overweight people need a diet, not thyroid treatment.

trying to pretend I really prefer listening to the music. Having a solicitious saleslady suggest that something a little *fuller* might be more flattering to my figure (or lack thereof). Having my mother tell me that the dress I finally, finally bought looks positively matronly. Periodically, these things all run together; I get depressed and upset enough about my excess fat to try and do something about it.

So, I'd start another diet. (I don't object at all to the word *diet*. Call it an eating program, a balanced nutritional pattern or whatever; it's diet. Why play with words?) Any diet is pretty easy for the first few days. I'm generally carried along on a wave of self-satisfaction, encouragement from others, and the pleasure of discovering that I do, after all, have will power and *can* lose weight. I think most people who want to lose weight know pretty much how they should eat. A good breakfast, sugar substitute in the coffee, one slice of toast, easy on the margarine. A salad, maybe some meat and fruit for lunch. Meat, fish, poultry, vegetables for dinner. No snacks, no desserts, etc. We've been taught it in school, heard of it on TV, read it in the *Ladies' Home Journal*. But, for me, again and again, knowing all this, it still hasn't worked.

But it *is* possible to lose weight successfully and not gain it back. If you're aware of the danger signals, you can take steps to counteract them:

1. Don't start on a diet without thinking it through. Go to a doctor on the chance that there *might* be a metabolic basis for your fat. Don't start on an impulse, because the momentum will not last long.

2. Pick a sensible diet and plan on something you can stay with for a long time. Could you really eat grapefruit for the rest of your life?

3. Be patient and try to take a long-range view. Aim for, say, five pounds in a month, one hundred pounds in two years. This, I think, is

the hardest part, but it's the only rational approach to take.

4. Have someone to talk to. Not your friends or coworkers, since they're interested, but generally pretty bored by endless talk of dieting. Go to a group meeting, or a doctor, or talk to people who've lost a lot of weight themselves. I've found them to be pretty sympathetic and encouraging listeners. NOTE: I've found that it's disastrous to go food shopping when you're at a low point moralewise. Everything looks *so* good! It's more expensive, and then you feel obligated to eat all that junk that you bought.

5. Find other ways to cheer yourself up. This is generally more time consuming and requires more thought than just going to the refrigerator. Whatever you pick (a walk, a bike ride, a museum, a tennis game, shopping) usually has the added benefit of involving at least minimal physical exertion.

6. If none of the above works, and you're really fed up (I think this is almost inevitable in any long diet), go ahead and indulge, but set a ceiling of five to ten pounds gained before you start again in earnest. In the overall picture this is lost time, but sometimes it is the only way. I know after a few days of indulging myself after months of dieting, I usually feel guilty and annoyed at myself and start back in again.

In summary, I find my two main problems in dieting are:

1. Impatience.

2. Feeling guilty and depressed. After about six months of consistent progress the impatience pretty much goes away. The guilty feelings

stay around as long as I go off and on any diet. I used to think I had absolutely no will power, no motivation, and couldn't finish something that I'd started. That's a pretty depressing opinion to have of yourself. But with long experience, I've realized that dieting is *hard*. Worth it, but hard. Slipping occasionally is permissible, as long as it's not too often and too far.

If dieting were easy, no one would be fat.

Reference and Comment

Suggestions for Further Reading

Some Useful Information

Glossary of Terms

Index

Reference and Comment

1. In California, for example, 2704 patients who came to the Kaiser-Permanente Medical Center in Oakland for a general checkup in 1977 had thyroid tests performed as part of their examination. This survey showed that 0.31 percent of those patients had unsuspected hypothyroidism, a total of 0.81 percent who were ill but didn't know it. Assuming a population of 220 million in the United States, there may be 1.8 million people who would benefit from treatment if they could be found. (L. V. dos Remedios et al., *Archives of Internal Medicine* 140 [1980]: 1045.)

2. The following table gives the approximate amounts of radiation that your thyroid and your body receive if you have a thyroid scan. We include all three radioactive isotopes (two forms of radioactive iodine and radioactive technetium) that are in common use in thyroid scanning laboratories. The differences in radiation dosage given by the different isotopes depend upon the amounts of energy that they deliver to body tissues as well as the length of time they remain in your body.

RADIOSIOTOPE	USUAL SCAN DOSE		RADIATION DELIVERED TO THYROID	RADIATION DELIVERED TO WHOLE BODY
[131]Iodine	30–60	microcuries	33–66 rads	0.014–0.028 rads
[123]Iodine	100–400	microcuries	1.1–4.4 rads	0.003–0.012 rads
[99m]Technetium	5,000–10,000	microcuries	1–2 rads	0.06–0.12 rads

(Adapted from E. L. Sanger et al., *Journal of Nuclear Medicine* 19 [1978]; 107.)

For comparison, x-rays made of your kidneys expose your body to a radiation dose of about 2 rads, and a barium enema performed to x-ray your large intestine exposes you to slightly more radiation. As you can see, only the thyroid dose from [131]Iodine is outside this general range of radiation reached by a variety of testing procedures in use today. The Nuclear Regulatory Commission recommends that no one exceed 5 rads whole-body radiation in one year, so we are within that "safe range." Even so, your physician will perform such tests only if the radiation exposure is justified by the potential value of the information so obtained.

3. Doctors in Sweden recently examined 10,133 patients from 12 to 25 years (mean 18 years) after they had had a ^{131}I radioiodine thyroid scan. There was no increased evidence of thyroid cancer among the scanned patients when compared with the population at large. (L. E. Holm et al., *Journal of the National Cancer Institute* 64 [1980]: 1055.)

4. Physicians have used radioactive iodine to treat and control overactive thyroids since 1939, and in the intervening years have not found this particular treatment to be associated with any increased risk of thyroid cancer. We do not know why this is so, but we suspect that the dose of radiation to the thyroid is so large (7,000–50,000 rads) that we somehow destroy the ability of those thyroid cells to become cancerous. Nevertheless, we continue to watch patients who have been treated in this manner, to be sure that cancers or other thyroid problems will not develop later in life.

5. D. S. Cooper, et al., *Annals of Internal Medicine* 98 [1983] 26.

6. Choosing the correct dose of radioactive iodine for each patient is difficult since the effect of ^{131}I depends on

many variables, most of which cannot be easily measured or anticipated:

   a. Size of the thyroid gland, or the amount of thyroid tissue to be treated.
   b. Percent uptake of the ^{131}I by the thyroid gland, which determines how much of the administered ^{131}I actually reaches the thyroid tissue.
   c. Length of time that the ^{131}I actually remains in the thyroid—the longer the time, the greater its effect on the thyroid tissue.
   d. Individual variation in sensitivity to ^{131}I, including such factors as the patient's age, prior antithyroid drug treatments, and the presence of other medications that might affect the patient's sensitivity to radioiodine.

In spite of these variables, radioactive iodine remains the treatment of choice for many hyperthyroid patients, most of whom experience excellent therapeutic results.

7. An early case report suggested that if propranolol was being given to a pregnant mother at the time of delivery, her baby might not breathe properly immediately after birth. (M. E. Tunstace, *British Journal of Anesthesia* 41 [1969]: 792.)

Another report indicated that long-term administration of this drug during pregnancy might be associated with a small placenta, poor fetal growth, and other depressive effects on the baby after birth, including a low blood sugar and slow pulse. (G. R. Gladstone et al. *Journal of Pediatrics* 86 [1975]: 962.)

Our present reluctance to use propranolol in pregnancy over long periods, and especially near the time of expected delivery, is based upon such reports. It is possible, however, that wider experience with the drug may show that it is not as harmful as these early reports suggest. If so, propranolol may assume a more important role in the management of hyperthyroidism in pregnancy.

8. The first suggestion that overactive thyroids of Graves' disease tend to fail in later years came in 1888, when physicians commented that patients with "exophthalmic goiter" sometimes developed "myxedema" (hypothyroidism) even though the only treatments for hyperthyroidism at that time were rest and supportive care. (*Transactions of the Clinical Society of London* 21, supplement [1888]: 180.) Other medical reports have supported this view and have appeared from time to time since then. For example, in 1928, Dr. John Eason wrote of his hypothyroid patients that they often had a history, years earlier, of apparent unrecognized hyperthyroidism, which included exophthalmos. (*Edinburgh Medical Journal* 39 [1932]: 507.)

9. L. C. Wood and S. H. Ingbar, *Journal of Clinical Investigation* 64 (1979): 1429.

10. This information comes from a remarkable survey in which British physicians carried out careful thyroid tests in one fifth of the inhabitants of the entire town of Whickham, a total of 2779 people. (W. M. G. Tunbridge et al., *Clinical Endocrinology* 7 [1977]:481.)

11. R. W. Rees-Jones et al., *Journal of the American Medical Association* 243 (1980): 549.

12. There is even a real possibility that Graves' disease and Hashimoto's disease represent different parts of a single thyroid disorder. They tend to run in the same families, and sometimes in the same patient there will be evidence of both conditions, when the clinical course and pathology of thyroid tissue are carefully examined. There are even reports of identical twins in which one twin had Graves' disease, the other Hashimoto's thyroiditis. Finally, as shown later in this chapter, patients with both conditions show the same tendencies to develop associated medical problems, such as diabetes mellitus and pernicious anemia.

13. In the early 1970s physicians at the University of Chicago examined 100 asymptomatic patients who had a history of head or neck radiation in childhood. Among these patients, the thyroid gland felt abnormal in 26. Of these 26 patients, 15 contained nodules that were felt possibly to be cancer. When these 15 were operated upon, 7 of the 15 glands (in 7 percent of the original 100 patients) contained cancer. Similarly, doctors at Michael Reese Hospital and Medical Center in Chicago have reviewed 1056 radiated patients. As with the University of Chicago findings, 27 percent of the patients had abnormal thyroid glands by examination or testing and cancer was found in about 6 percent of the total group of 1056 patients. These figures contrast with a national cancer survey carried out in 1969 to 1971, which indicated that the annual incidence of thyroid cancer in the general population is one per 37,000 or 0.004 percent. Reports such as these suggest that we are dealing with a major public health problem, and accordingly, in 1976 the U.S. Department of Health, Education, and Welfare sponsored a conference on the subject of radiation-associated thyroid cancer. The 150 physicians and other health professionals who attended this conference reviewed the problem from many points of view based upon experience all over the United States. They estimated the risk of thyroid cancers in such people to be somewhat lower and gave the following example. "If 25 years ago the thyroid glands of 100 people were exposed to 300 rads each . . . about two will have developed thyroid cancer and nine will have thyroid glands in which there only benign nodules." The term *300 rads* refers to a specific dose of radiation and is in the range received by the thyroid gland of many of the patients we were talking about.

14. This information comes from a study of children who received radiation in the Marshall Islands in 1954, when fallout from an atomic explosion at Bikini accidentally blew over these islands due to an unexpected change in

wind direction. When the inhabitants of these islands were examined by doctors in 1976, more benign thyroid nodules were found in individuals who had been under ten years of age when exposed to the radiation than in those over ten years of age in 1954. Specifically, 18 out of 23 inhabitants who had been under ten years of age had developed nodules in contrast to 6 out of 45 who had been over ten years of age at exposure and subsequently developed thyroid nodules. The incidence of thyroid cancer was about 5 percent in both groups.

15. Some physicians recommend that all patients who have ever been radiated in childhood should take thyroid tablets to minimize the likelihood of thyroid cancer developing later in life. However the data about this point is controversial enough that a definitive statement as to the value of thyroxine treatment cannot be made at this time. Therefore, most doctors do not recommend "suppressive" thyroid hormone therapy routinely for radiated patients.

16. In a nonpregnant woman, a TRH test, which is described in detail in Chapter 4, is a safe and easy way to tell if hyperthyroidism is present if the diagnosis is in doubt. This test is not usually performed during pregnancy, however, because it requires that the patient be given an injection of the hormone TRH. Although TRH has not yet been approved for use in pregnancy, there is no evidence that it is likely to be harmful to the mother or her unborn child.

17. When we say that one in 70 babies born to hyperthyroid mothers will be hyperthyroid too, we are referring to a medical study of newborn children that was published in 1962. In our experience this problem is *very* rare. Perhaps a more modern study of the same problem would show that it is less common today.

18. If a severely hypothyroid baby is not treated with thyroid hormone before it is three months old, permanent mental and physical retardation may occur. Unfortunately, such babies often do not look sick at birth, and typical features of hypothyroidism (including sleepiness and lethargy, a hoarse low cry, and puffy skin) may not become apparent until after the mother has taken the baby home from the hospital. Therefore, since we can prevent children with hypothyroidism from developing serious permanent disabilities by early thyroid hormone treatment, physicians throughout most of North America as well as in many other countries now test *all* newborn babies for hypothyroidism by measuring their thyroid hormone level in a sample of umbilical cord blood. Once the condition is recognized, treatment is straightforward. The mother gives her baby thyroid hormone by mouth once a day along with his or her regular feeding.

19. It has been estimated that a breast-feeding baby might receive from 10 to 100 microcuries of radioactive iodine in the first day after its mother is treated with a usual dose of 5 millicuries of radioactive iodine. Each microcurie that the baby absorbs could deliver 30 rads of radiation effect to the infant's thyroid—a theoretical maximum dose of 300 rads. Most physicians would agree that that amount of irradiation to an infant's immature thyroid would significantly increase the likelihood that the child would someday develop thyroid nodules or thyroid cancer (see also Chapter 12).

20. We used to believe that stillbirths and birth defects were more common among infants born to mothers with hypothyroidism compared with infants born to mothers with healthy thyroid glands. However, recent medical reports suggest that this may not be the case. Despite this more optimistic outlook for the children of mothers with undiscovered hypothyroidism, if you are found to be hypothyroid in pregnancy *all* physicians would prefer

to treat that condition with thyroid hormone rather than take *any* risk of your child's developing any problem due to your condition.

21. The reasons that it is no longer possible to make a meaningful list of the iodine content of foods are well-expressed by the following excerpt from a book about nutrition:

> The iodine content of milk, other dairy products, and egg varies with the composition of the animals' food. The amount of iodine in bread varies with the mixing process used. One slice of bread made by the continuous mix process will supply the daily iodine requirement (100 micrograms of iodine), while one slice made by the batch process contains very little.
> ... Since growing plants pick up iodine when it is present in the soil, plant foods vary widely in iodine content according to the soil in which they are grown... Thus plant foods grown near seacoasts and in our Southern states contain more iodine than those grown in the Great Lakes area or other regions where the surface soil is low in iodine. For these reasons it is impossible to list the iodine content of foods in tables of food composition or to estimate the amount in the dietary pattern. (H. S. Mitchell et al., *Nutrition in Health and Disease* 16th ed. [Philadelphia: J. B. Lippincott Co., 1976].)

A balanced diet that avoids kelp should be enough to prevent an unhealthy dietary iodine excess except in most unusual circumstances.

Suggestions for Further Reading

1. OTHER BOOKS FOR PATIENTS AND THE GENERAL PUBLIC

- Baskin, H. Jack. *How Your Thyroid Works*. For copies send $1.50 to: Dr. Baskin, Florida Thyroid and Endocrine Clinic, 2921 N. Orange Avenue, Orlando, Florida 32804. (The price includes postage.)
- Bayliss, R. I. S. *Thyroid Disease, The Facts*. New York. Oxford University Press, 1982.
- Hamburger, Joel I. *The Thyroid Gland: A Book for Thyroid Patients*. (Third Edition, 1985.) For copies send $5.00 to:

  Joel Hamburger, M.D.
  2988 Telegraph Road
  Southfield, Michigan 48034

2. MEDICAL TEXTBOOKS ABOUT THE THYROID

- De Groot, Leslie J., and John B. Stanbury. *The Thyroid and Its Diseases*. (Fifth Edition). New York. John Wiley & Sons, Inc., 1984.
- DeVisscher, Michael, Editor. *The Thyroid Gland*. (Comprehensive Endocrinology Series). New York. Raven Press, 1980.
- Hamburger, Joel I. *Management of Thyroid Pa-

tients. (Second Edition, 1985.) For copies, write to Dr. Hamburger at the address given above. Prices are: Volume I, $32.00; and Volume II, $36.00.

- Werner, Sidney C., and Sidney H. Ingbar, Editors. *The Thyroid, A Fundamental and Clinical Text*. (Fourth Edition). New York. Harper and Row, 1978. (A new edition is due in 1986.)

3. GENERAL ENDOCRINOLOGY INFORMATION

- Greenspan, Francis S., and Peter H. Forsham. *Basic and Clinical Endocrinology*. Los Altos. Lange Medical Publications, 1983.
- Wilson, Jean D., and Daniel W. Foster. *Williams' Textbook of Endocrinology*. (Seventh Edition). Philadelphia. W. B. Saunders Co., 1985.

For information about the thyroid, most individuals should begin with one of the books in category 1. Books in categories 2 and 3 are generally more costly and are written for health professionals. However, if your library has an "interlibrary loan service," your librarian should be able to borrow a copy for you if you desire.

Thyroid Organizations You Might Want to Know About:

Information For Physicians

The American Thyroid Association
Secretary Colum A. Gorman M.D., Ph.D.
Department of Endocrinology,
The Mayo Clinic
200 First St. SW
Rochester, MN 55901

Information For Patients and Other Health Professionals

The Thyroid Foundation of America, Inc.
630 WANG Ambulatory Care Center
Massachusetts General Hospital
Boston, MA 02114

The Thyroid Foundation of Canada
CD/PO Box 1643
Kingston, Ontario
Canada K7l 5C8

Some Useful Information

Abbreviations

T_3—Triiodothynine   }Thyroid hormones
T_4—Thyroxine

T_3 **suppression test**—a thyroid test in which a patient takes T_3 tablets in an attempt to reduce thyroid function

T_3 **resin uptake**—a blood test done to evaluate the degree to which thyroid hormones are bound to blood proteins

Free T_4 Index (T_7)—a mathematical calculation derived by multiplying the $T_4 \times T_3$ resin uptake that is done in order to evaluate thyroid function

TSH—thyroid stimulating hormone

TRH—TSH releasing hormone, used for testing pituitary-thyroid relationship

RAI—radioactive iodine, used for testing and treating the thyroid

RAIU—radioactive iodine uptake, a thyroid function test

^{131}I, ^{123}I—radioactive isotopes of iodine

^{99m}Tc—radioactive technetium, a radioactive isotope sometimes used in place of radioiodine in the performance of thyroid uptake and scans

NORMAL LABORATORY VALUES

Normal values vary considerably from laboratory to laboratory and therefore tests can only be interpreted if the normal ranges for the laboratory where they were performed are known. A given range of normal (e.g., T_4: 4–12 mcg/dl) means that 95 percent of a normal population of people will have T_4 values within those limits. The normal ranges for common thyroid blood tests at the MGH Thyroid Unit are as follows:

T_4: 4–12 mcg/dl (micrograms/deciliter)
T_3: 75–195/dl (nanograms/deciliter)
T_3 Resin Uptake: 25–35%
Free T_4 Index: 1–4
TSH: 0.5–5.0/mU (microunits/milliliter)

DRUGS USED BY THYROID PATIENTS

Thyroid Hormones
    thyroxine (T_4)—Levothroid, Synthroid, Eltroxin
    triiodothyronine (T_3)—Cytomel
    desiccated thyroid—powdered animal thyroid
    thyroglobulin—Proloid
    T_3-T_4 mixtures—Euthyroid, Thyrolar
Antithyroid Drugs
    propylthiouracil—often just referred to as "PTU"
    methimazole—Tapazole
    carbimazole—similar to Tapazole and used in England and Europe
Drugs that block the action of thryoid hormones on body tissues
    propranolol—Inderal
Iodine Preparations
    potassium iodide
    saturated solution of potassium iodide—may be referred to also as "SSKI"
    Lugol's solution

Miscellaneous drugs mentioned in this book
 radioactive iodine—used to test and treat the thyroid
 psoralins—used to treat vitiligo
 Vitamin B_{12}—used to treat pernicious anemia (combined systems disease)
Beta-adrenergic-blocking drugs that block the action of thyroid hormones in body tissues
 Short-acting:
 propranolol—Inderal
 Long-acting:
 acebutalol—Sectral
 atenolol—Tenormin
 metaprolol—Lopressor
 nadolol—Corgard
 propranalol (long-acting)—Inderal-LA
 timolol—Blocadren

 }

 Thyroid hormones

Glossary of Terms

Addison's disease—a disease caused by failure of the adrenal glands.

agranulocytosis—an uncommon blood disorder in which certain white blood cells known as granulocytes disappear from the blood. It may occur as an allergic reaction to an antithyroid drug.

alopecia—hair loss.

alopecia areata—a patchy hair loss sometimes found in patients with Graves' disease or Hashimoto's thyroiditis.

anemia—a low red blood cell count.

antibody—a protein substance produced by the body against something known as an *antigen*. Antithyroid antibodies appear in the blood of patients with certain thyroid conditions and seem to have a role in stimulating or inflaming the thyroid gland.

antithyroid drug—a drug that acts upon the thyroid to decrease its function.

basal metabolic rate (BMR)—a test that measures the amount of oxygen used by the body. Formerly a common thyroid function test, it has now largely been replaced by more precise tests, which measure hormone levels directly.

beta adrenergic blocking drugs—drugs that are used to block the action of thyroid hormones on body tissues (atenolol and propanolol are common examples).

biopsy—an operation in which a small sample of tissue is obtained for examination.

calcitonin—a protein that may increase in the blood in

association with a form of thyroid cancer known as *medullary carcinoma*.

carcinoma—cancer. *Follicular*, *papillary*, *Hürthle cell*, and *medullary carcinoma* are types of thyroid cancer, so named for their appearance or the kind of thyroid cell type from which they arise. *Anaplastic* carcinoma is the most serious form of thyroid cancer and is made up of immature or undifferentiated thyroid cells.

carrier proteins—proteins that transport hormones through the blood stream.

cerebral cortex—the outermost nerve tissue on and near the surface of the brain.

chronic lymphocytic thyroiditis (Hashimoto's disease)—long-standing low-grade inflammation of the thyroid that lead to thyroid failure (hypothyroidism) in later life.

cold nodule—a nonfunctioning lump in the thyroid gland.

combined systems disease—pernicious anemia. The term actually includes disorders of the blood (anemia) as well as the nervous system (numb hands and feet and loss of balance) that occur if there is a deficiency of Vitamin B_{12}.

cortisone—an important steroid hormone made by the adrenal gland.

cretinism—a severe form of hypothyroidism that begins before birth and causes severe disturbances of growth and development.

cutting needle biopsy—a biopsy performed with a sharp hollow needle by means of which a core of tissue is obtained for examination.

cyst—a fluid-filled lump.

decompression—an operation done to relieve pressure. In thyroid disease it usually refers to surgery done to reduce pressure within the bony orbit (eye socket) of a patient with protruding eyes.

DeQuervain's disease—subacute thyroiditis.

dessicated thyroid—dried animal thyroid tissue that has been made into thyroid hormone tablets.

diffuse toxic goiter (Graves' disease)—hyperthyroidism caused by a generalized overactivity of the entire thyroid gland.

dysfunction—abnormal function. The term *thyroid dysfunction* usually refers to an overactive or underactive thyroid gland.

dyslexia—certain types of learning difficulties that are inherited and not due to physical or emotional handicaps.

exophthalmos—protrusion of one or both eyes. The most common cause is Graves' disease.

fine needle aspiration—a biopsy done with a small needle through which a few cells are obtained for examination.

galactorrhea—milk in the breasts at a time other than while nursing a baby.

goiter—an enlarged thyroid from any cause.

> *multinodular goiter*: a goiter containing more than one lump.
>
> *nodular goiter*: one containing one or more lumps.
>
> *nontoxic goiter*: a goiter that has not caused hyperthyroidism.
>
> *simple goiter*: one without lumps
>
> *diffuse goiter*: one without lumps.

Graves' disease—diffuse toxic goiter.

Hashimoto's disease—chronic lymphocytic thyroiditis.

hormone—a chemical made by a gland, such as the thyroid, adrenal, or pancreas. Hormones may travel to some other part of the body to product an effect.

hot nodule (Plummer's disease)—an overactive thyroid lump.

hyperthyroidism—a condition caused by too much thyroid hormone in the body.

hypothalamus—part of the brain that controls the pituitary gland's function.

hypothyroidism—a condition caused by too little thyroid hormone in the body.

> *Primary* hypothyroidism is caused by disease within the thyroid.

Secondary hypothyroidism is caused by pituitary gland trouble.

Tertiary hypothyroidism is caused by diseases within the hypothalamus.

inflammation—tissue changes that occur in response to injury. Thyroid inflammation (thyroiditis) may lead to scarring hypothyroidism.

intrinsic factor—a chemical substance that helps us to absorb Vitamin B_{12} from food. A lack of intrinsic factor may lead to pernicious anemia.

iodine—the chemical element in our diet with which thyroid hormone is made.

isthmus—the part of the thyroid gland between the two lobes.

kelp—seaweed, a health food that contains iodine.

lymphocyte—a type of white blood cell that makes antibodies. Lymphocytes are found in increased numbers in the thyroid glands of patients with thyroiditis.

myxedema—a term used for severe hypothyroidism.

neonatal hyperthyroidism—an overactive thyroid in a newborn baby.

neutrophil—a kind of white blood cell (also called a *granulocyte*) that helps to control infections. Neutrophils may decrease in number as part of an allergic reaction to an antithyroid drug.

nodule—a lump.

optic neuropathy—inflammation of the nerve of the eye that occurs rarely in patients with Graves' disease.

parathyroid glands—glands near the thyroid that help control the calcium level.

periodic paralysis—episodic weakness. It may be caused by potassium deficiency in occasional patients with hyperthyroidism.

pernicious anemia—a low red blood cell count caused by a lack of Vitamin B_{12}.

pituitary gland—a gland at the base of the brain that controls the functions of the thyroid and other glands, including the adrenals, ovaries, and testes.

Plummer's disease—hyperthyroidism caused by one or more overactive thyroid nodules.

pretibial myxedema—a reddish thickening of the skin over the front of the legs that may occur in Graves' disease.

protein-bound iodine concentration (PBI)—the amount of iodine that is chemically attached to protein in the blood. Once a common thyroid test, it has been replaced by more specific measurements of the thyroid hormones themselves.

pyramidal lobe—a projection of thyroid tissue extending upward from the isthmus of the thyroid gland.

rad—*r*adiation *a*bsorbed *d*ose—a measure of the amount of radiation delivered to tissue.

radioactive iodine (radioiodine)—a form of iodine used to test and treat thyroid conditions.

radioactive iodine uptake test—a thyroid test in which measurement is made of the percent of swallowed radioiodine that is taken up by the thyroid. The test is usually performed 24 hours after administration of the radioiodine.

radioactive scan—a picture of the thyroid made with radioiodine.

receptor—proteins in cells to which thyroid and other hormones bind, thereby initiating the effects of the hormones.

recurrent laryngeal nerves—nerves that supply the vocal chords and may be injured during thyroid surgery.

roentgen—a measurement of the amount of radiation delivered from a radiation source.

Schilling test—a test performed to measure Vitamin B_{12} absorption from the stomach.

sedimentation rate— a blood test measuring the speed at which red blood cells settle in a thin tube, which is used as a way of detecting the presence of inflammation in the body.

spontaneously resolving hyperthyroidism hyperthyroid—ism that goes away by itself without specific treatment. It may occur more than once in a given patient.

spontaneous remission—the disappearance of a disease without specific treatment.

subacute thyroiditis (DeQuervain's disease)—thyroid inflammation associated with pain and swelling of the thyroid gland.

thyroglobulin—a complex protein molecule in which thyroid hormones are stored within the thyroid gland. The concentration of thyroglobulin in blood is increased in some patients with thyroid cancer as well as with certain other conditions.

thyroidectomy—surgical removal of the thyroid gland.

thyroiditis—inflammation or infection of the thyroid gland.

thyroid stimulating hormone (TSH)—a pituitary gland hormone that increases thyroid function.

thyrotoxicosis—hyperthyroidism from any cause.

thyroxine (T_4)—one of the thyroid hormones.

transducer—an instrument that changes energy from one form to another. For example, in an ultrasound test, a transducer changes sound waves into a thyroid picture.

triiodothyronine (T_3)—one of the thyroid hormones.

T_3 resin uptake test—a blood test used to tell how much thyroid hormone is free to act upon body tissue and how much is bound to protein in an inactive form.

tumor—a lump. A *benign* tumor is harmless, a *malignant* tumor is cancerous.

ultrasound thyroid picture—a picture of the thyroid made by using sound waves in a manner similar to radar.

vitiligo—a harmless condition in which white spots appear on the skin. Vitiligo is found in patients with certain thyroid problems, as well as in some people who have no obvious thyroid abnormality.

Index

ABOUT THE AUTHORS

The three authors of *Your Thyroid* bring strong research and clinical backgrounds to this valuable book for both general readers and thyroid patients. The first edition was written while the three authors were practicing together in the Thyroid Unit of the Massachusetts General Hospital in Boston. They still share the common interests in patient and public education expressed in this volume, and keep in close touch with one another even though Dr. Ridgway is now Head of the Endocrine Division at the University of Colorado Health Sciences Center, and Dr. Cooper has gone to the Sinai Hospital of Baltimore, where he is Associate Head of The Endocrinology and Metabolism Division and Associate Chief of the Thyroid Unit at the Johns Hopkins Hospital.

All three are actively involved in the American Thyroid Association as well as the Thyroid Foundation of America. This volume attests to their continuing commitment to educating and supporting thyroid patients and health professionals and increasing public awareness about thyroid problems.